# The Modern Guide to GP Consulting: Six S for Success

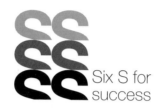

Six S for success

**ALEX WATSON**

*General Practitioner*
*Ashtead and Leatherhead, Surrey*

and

**DAVID GILLESPIE**

*Actor, Writer, Producer*
*Corporate Coach and Co-founder, The Speechworks*

*Forewords by*

**PROFESSOR ABDOL TAVABIE**

*Dean of Postgraduate GP Education*
*Health Education Kent, Surrey and Sussex*

and

**SIR EDWARD CLAY**

*Associate Director*
*Centre for Political and Diplomatic Studies*
*Westminster, London*

Radcliffe Publishing
London • New York

**Radcliffe Publishing Ltd**
St Mark's House
Shepherdess Walk
London N1 7LH
United Kingdom

www.radcliffehealth.com

British Library Cataloguing in Publication Data

A catalogue record for this book is available from the British Library.

ISBN-13: 978 190936 898 9

The paper used for the text pages of this book is FSC® certified. FSC (The Forest Stewardship Council®) is an international network to promote responsible management of the world's forests.

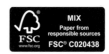

Illustrations on pp 10, 13, 29, 31, 42, 49, 57, 59, 70, 78, 89 and 95 produced by Ian Wilson, wearemash.com

Typeset by Darkriver Design, Auckland, New Zealand
Printed and bound by Hobbs the Printers, Totton, Hants, UK

# Contents

# Foreword by Professor Abdol Tavabie

Medical professionals have a number of characteristics in common. Communication is especially important as it is the basis of the special relationship with those whom we serve. Communication is an integral part of our work in the health service, and essential in delivering patient-centred care. Our ability to listen, to think and respond sensitively and effectively to our patients and their relatives, and to our team members who are responsible for the delivery of services, are crucial skills and should be in the forefront of our minds.

*The Modern Guide to GP Consulting: Six S for Success* provides a fresh, sound and simple framework to improve the way we communicate with our patients. In so doing, we enrich our relationships, enhance our influence and expand our capacity to deliver high-quality patient services.

The book begins by defining the significance of communication skills and identifies a series of tasks to be undertaken. The approach is as useful for expert professionals as for novices in identifying the real issues which are relevant to our patients, as well as taking care of ourselves in emotionally charged consultations.

The collaboration of Watson and Gillespie – the doctor and the actor – has produced an original and insightful guide to the role of the general practitioner (GP). They describe vividly the GP as witness of their patients' symptoms and concerns, and as advisor on alleviating their suffering. They illustrate with effective narratives the way in which we can develop our powers of observation, communication and self-awareness.

This book is clear and easy to follow in language that all of us understand. It is an invaluable source of refreshment, inspiration, education and reflection. I recommend it to all clinicians.

**Professor Abdol Tavabie**
**Dean of Postgraduate GP Education**
**Health Education Kent, Surrey and Sussex**
*September 2013*

# Foreword by Sir Edward Clay

A link between medical general practice and diplomacy isn't obvious. So, as a former diplomat – and patient of British and foreign doctors in different cultures – I was slightly surprised to warm so readily to this book. Its cheerful presentation of practical advice on how to manage relationships is useful not only for doctors, but for anyone required to engage intimately on a professional level with people to whom they are not personally close.

Interpersonal relations are at the heart of diplomacy. So every chapter in this book speaks to me. Ambassadors see all manner of people, well disposed or unfriendly, and are often suspicious about the encounter. A useful meeting requires a sound basis in human relations, clarity about the agenda, effective communication between the parties, agreement about what is to be done and commitment to do it.

Cultural factors are key. They are the context of all human transactions, everywhere. Heidi's story (*see* p. 32) is a moving illustration of this. For diplomats, as for doctors, good communication begins with listening,

With listening goes observing. The diplomat, like the doctor, whether trying to persuade or to negotiate, listens to the words and watches the body language of the other party. Reject distractions by a screen, or a brief or notes: the discussion requires 101% focus. Prepare before, write it up afterwards; take only the briefest note during the discussion, lest you lose the flow or a key point. You waste your precious face time if you don't look your patient in the eye.

In diplomatic negotiation, both sides should have the same understanding of what they've agreed. Doctors have short consultations. You want the patient to emerge convinced that your advice will benefit his or her health; you and she or he need to agree on the best course to follow, and be equally committed to it. Speak clearly and unambiguously.

First impressions are important. They get proper emphasis here. If people approach a meeting with a GP or an ambassador in a negative frame of mind, fearing being talked down to, being treated as an inconvenience, or whatever, the meeting may fail.

One idea an ambassador might offer: standing up and shaking hands with callers is the way much of the world still behaves. In some cultures the hand may be placed over the heart instead. Such a greeting powerfully indicates common humanity, goodwill and good faith: it levels the richest and the poorest, the powerful and the powerless, and works with strangers, friends and acquaintances.

The vanishing handshake culture in Britain is a loss. Even for GPs, groaning under time pressures, there are practical advantages: standing and shaking hands creates that necessary airlock between patients, breaks the tyranny of the screen and allows the doctor to observe the caller before they start their discussion.

A clear interest in your patient is the biggest compliment a doctor can pay; it repays the effort. It begins with the non-verbal statement that the handshake conveys.

Medicine owes a lot to Scots. So does poetry to Burns. Perhaps ambassadors, doctors and patients could remember:

> O wad some Pow'r the giftie gie us
> To see oursels as others see us!
> It wad frae mony a blunder free us,
> An' foolish notion.

Insight and self-awareness matter most.

This book is a goldmine of robust good sense for doctors. We now need a guide to being a good patient.

**Sir Edward Clay**
**Associate Director**
**Centre for Political and**
**Diplomatic Studies**
**Westminster, London**
*September 2013*

# About the authors

**Alex** is a GP in Ashtead and Leatherhead, Surrey. He graduated from University College London with a psychology degree and studied medicine at the University of Leeds. He completed his GP training in Epsom, having worked previously in Bristol and Reading. Alex is currently a GP trainer and has successfully supported numerous underperforming trainees through their Clinical Skills Assessment, an essential part of the membership examination for the Royal College of General Practitioners. He was a programme director for the Epsom GP Vocational Training Scheme from 2004 to 2009, during which time he completed a postgraduate certificate in medical education. He is co-author of *ENT in Primary Care*, a handbook for primary care practitioners, and he has led local community ear, nose and throat services since 2006 in collaboration with specialist consultant colleagues from four different acute medical trusts. Alex is passionate about communication and education, which he promotes through each of his various roles as a doctor.

**David** is an actor, writer, producer, corporate coach and co-founder of The Speechworks (www.thespeechworks.co.uk). As an actor David has performed in theatres all over the world and in London's West End – he has appeared in numerous films and TV programmes and he led the cast of BBC Two's *Operation Good Guys* to win both Gold and Silver Roses at the Montreux TV Festival. He is the co-author of three books on communications skills and one play, *Sleep No More*, a supernatural thriller, co-written with Colin Wakefield. His latest book, *How to be Interesting*, co-written with Mark Warren, has featured regularly in WHSmith's bestseller list. With The Speechworks he provides communication and presentation skills coaching for some of the world's most senior business figures. David is a much sought-after speaker to the international business community and is regularly asked to give comment on the communication skills of our political leaders on such programmes as the BBC's *Worldwide News* and *Newsnight*.

# Note to the reader

For reasons of confidentiality we have changed the names of the story contributors, and in some instances parts of the narrative, but the story contributors' thoughts and feelings remain faithfully reflected.

*We would like to dedicate this book to Chaz, Biz, Ellie, Niamh, Bella, Gabriella and Saskia, who always have a good story to share and who help keep us sane.*

# Introduction

*The art of medicine consists in amusing the
patient while nature cures the disease.*

Voltaire

There is much to be considered from Voltaire's humorous remark. The doctor–
patient relationship is probably the most talked-about and explored relationship
in both reality and fiction. There have possibly been more television programmes
made about doctors, nurses, patients, surgeries and hospitals than any other subject.
This is because the medical profession touches everyone. We begin our relationship
with medicine before we leave the womb and we continue interacting with it until
the day we die. How doctors and patients relate to each other will always be up for
debate. To listen, think and respond sensitively and effectively are essential skills
for anyone to have, whatever his or her business. In the medical profession, it is
vital that these abilities are active at all times. To be attuned to the needs, desires
and concerns of others plays a huge role in managing the well-being of patients,
their relatives and their friends. It is crucial these skills are always at the forefront
of the medic's toolkit. It is all too easy to treat the physical ailments and ignore the
psychological issues that may also be an integral part of the problems themselves.

*Six S for Success* is a simple and straightforward guide that we believe any doctor can use to improve the way they communicate with their patients. For many
years, general practitioners (GPs) have placed great emphasis and importance
on consultation skills especially within their training schemes. Medical schools
are placing increasing value on these skills, regardless of what specialty a doctor
chooses to pursue in the future.

Using our six Ss – **Status, Story, Summarising, Sharing, Securing and Sanity**
– we will provide you with a framework to improve your chances of successful
consultations. So let us briefly outline what we will be covering in each 'S'.

1. **Status**: this is how people perceive us and how we want to be perceived. How
   patients perceive their doctors may affect the quality of their encounter. We
   will explore how a patient's experience can shape outcomes. First impressions

count, so let us help you get it right first time. Much is made of 'building a good rapport', but how exactly do you do this with each patient, considering the time pressures and other demands upon you?

2. **Story**: storytelling is our most basic form of communication. It is how most of us convey our thoughts, feelings and ideas. So let your patients tell their story. Hear what has brought them to see you *today*. Doctors have their lists of questions to ask, attempting to clarify suspected diagnoses, as well as excluding serious pathology. How do you get the right balance of questioning and listening? We will explore six different types of listening, as well as examine our verbal and non-verbal methods of communication, and how we integrate and employ our skills effectively.

3. **Summarising**: this is a well-recognised but much underused technique that allows doctors to feed back what they have heard and understood from the patient. It is also a great tool to focus on what exactly the patient is concerned about, which doctors can then acknowledge. How often do you summarise during each of your consultations? We will discuss the wider benefits of summarising to both doctors and patients, which should help to address the more managerial aspects of consultations.

4. **Sharing**: usually the pinnacle of the consultation is sharing the options and deciding on what the most appropriate action (or inaction) should be next. For this is what your encounter with your patient has been building towards, from the moment they decided to seek your medical advice. Yet, this is easier said than done. Why should doctors not just tell patients what to do? We should, after all, come from a position of greater knowledge and expertise. We will explain not only why sharing the responsibility with your patients results in them being more engaged in their care, and more compliant with treatment plans, but also how it allows doctors to share the burden of risk.

5. **Securing**: securing the consultation is about ensuring the doctor–patient encounter reaches a clear and safe conclusion. It involves both the doctor and the patient clarifying what their roles are, and will be, in any further ongoing care. In a litigious world the stakes are rarely higher than in the medical profession. GPs in particular can feel vulnerable, practising more in isolation without a team of colleagues or more immediate investigations at hand to call on to aid diagnosis. There is a risk that doctors practise medicine defensively, which is not always in the patient's best interest. We will describe further how, by taking a balanced approach and including your patient (or his or her advocate), this can improve results and lead to a safe and agreeable conclusion.

6. **Sanity**: this covers not only the doctor's need to refocus before seeing his or her next patient but also how the doctor survives and ideally enjoys his or her role in the longer term. Clinical encounters can be challenging, intense and emotionally demanding. Each patient will expect 100% of your attention and expertise. How do you shed any 'baggage' from previous consultations before entering the next? You would not expect a surgeon who has just finished operating on one patient to start on the next without re-scrubbing and re-gowning. Why should it be any different within our consultations, regardless of the specialty? As privileged a profession as medicine can be, it is clear that many doctors find the responsibility and intensity of the job affects their own well-being, with a high risk of burnout. We will explore ways of keeping sane, where patient demand and financial pressures are a factor.

So there you have our six Ss:

**Status – Story – Summarising – Sharing – Securing – Sanity**.

We do not wish to be prescriptive and we recognise that different doctors have different working styles. However, we believe there are some basic fundamental principles that we can all apply to help with our patient encounters. While most of this book is aimed at individual doctors, we also acknowledge the role that a practice or organisation plays in enhancing or detracting from patient interaction.

Is medicine more of a science or an art? We believe it involves the balance of being analytical and intuitive. Our unusual pairing as co-authors is an interesting one. While Watson's role as a doctor has been to observe symptoms, diagnose and treat, Gillespie's job as an actor has been to observe behaviour and reproduce it. Collaboration on this book has been an enlightening journey for us both, and we believe that our separate areas of expertise have combined well to create new thinking on a subject that will always be under the microscope. So, if you would like to explore more and improve your 'bedside manner', read on.

# 1

# Status

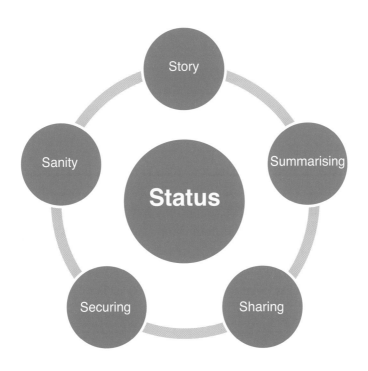

*It is only the shallow people who do not judge by appearances.*

Oscar Wilde

*At a round table there is no dispute about place.*

Italian proverb

# What is Status?

The sort of status we are referring to in this chapter has nothing to do with power, position, hierarchy, wealth, social standing or any of the words we might usually associate with the word 'status'. It's about perception: how we perceive people, how other people perceive us and how we want to be perceived. Status is physical, vocal and emotional. On a status scale of 1–10 we need to be hitting the middle status ground of 5–7 every time. We don't want to appear aloof, arrogant or snappy (10), but nor do we want to timidly apologise for ourselves (1). Mid-level status is strong and effective. It shows us to be accessible, warm and approachable, and it allows the patient to feel a sense of trust, confidence and safety.

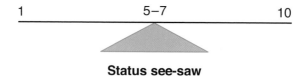

**Status see-saw**

You will notice that 'Status' appears at the centre of all of the Six S for Success diagrams in this book. This is because status touches all of the five other Ss – status is inextricably linked to them. When we become conscious of adopting the appropriate level of status for all of our communication, we begin to see positive changes in the way we address others and how we are perceived by them.

In this chapter, we will **explore the different levels of status – good and bad – and identify where we need to be on the status scale to get the best from our consultations**.

# Story 1: Showing an interest

*There are only two forces that unite men – fear and interest.*

Napoleon Bonaparte

There are few other professions more trusted than doctors. Our patients confide and share with us some of their most intimate thoughts and feelings, as well as their physical ailments. They expect their doctor to be caring, discreet, understanding, eager to help and interested. How would you feel if any of the words in the previous sentence did not feature in your patients' perceptions of you as their doctor? Heather describes her first experience with her new GP.

> Having recently joined a new surgery, my family and I were assigned to our new GP. I had no idea who she was or what she was like but I was soon to find out. I had a problem with my scalp, which itched and the skin was flaking, so I made an appointment to see her. When I knocked on her door I heard a loud and rather sharp-toned voice: 'Yes – come in!' As I entered the room the voice muttered for me to take a seat. After a few moments she asked what my problem was. When I had finished telling her about my scalp, she looked away from her computer screen, for the first time since I had entered the room, peered very briefly at the top of my head, went back to the screen and dashed off a prescription, which I took from her and left the room, still having had no eye contact or a pleasantry of any sort. I felt angry. I felt like she had no interest in me. It seemed that she didn't care. I wanted to complain but I didn't. I simply asked that my family be assigned to a different doctor, as I could not bear to think of my children being treated in that way.
>
> Heather, 38-year-old account manager

Heather experienced a doctor demonstrating a high level of status physically, vocally and emotionally. This began with a high vocal status (something we will explore in more depth later in this chapter), which immediately put her on edge. The lack of eye contact or any pleasantry heightened Heather's perception that this doctor had little personal interest in her. The emotional impact was profound.

This situation could quite easily have been very different. The doctor could have used a lighter vocal tone when asking Heather to come in. She could have looked up from her screen and greeted her more warmly, such as 'How can I help you today?' Heather might also have felt better about the consultation if the doctor had engaged her more by enquiring what she thought about the problem and whether she had experienced any previous episodes or treatment.

This story raises an interesting question of whether doctors should 'call' or 'collect' their patients. It is very much an individual matter and there are advantages to both. You may save a little time 'calling' your next patient in, giving you an opportunity to view his or her medical records, but what is the patient's experience? By 'collecting' the patient, you are initiating a rapport before the patient arrives in your room, and the added benefit of watching him or her walk in may provide you with valuable observations – mobility, gait, posture, breathing and general demeanour – all clues that aid in diagnosis.

# Story 2: We're all in this together

*Coming together is a beginning; keeping together
is progress; working together is success.*

Henry Ford

How often do you consider the impact that other staff and colleagues have on your patients? How do your patients perceive the quality of care offered by your organisation? For many, the patient experience starts the moment they pick up the phone to make contact with their doctor's surgery. If there is any fear about how they will be addressed or treated, be it over the phone or in person when they arrive for an appointment, then any existing worry and stress is likely to increase. Patient care is an ensemble piece. It requires everyone concerned in the process to be on the same status page and to be perceived in a favourable manner. Alan shares an experience he had at the reception of his doctor's surgery.

> I don't make many visits to my GP, so whenever I do the experience tends to be clear and sticks in my mind. I was recently at the surgery's reception trying to straighten out a problem with my daughter's medication. The receptionist helping me had gone to see the doctor who wrote the prescription. A young girl of about 16 or 17, a similar age to my daughter, was standing beside me being 'helped' by the other receptionist on duty. The girl was confused and wasn't able to articulate well or make herself properly understood. The situation clearly needed a little patience and understanding but she wasn't getting any. Although the girl had no problem with her hearing, the receptionist chose to raise her voice to her in an extremely condescending manner and punctuated what she said with heavy sighs of exasperation. This did nothing to help the young girl, who simply became more flustered. The receptionist then looked at me, gave a loud 'tut', raised her eyes to the ceiling and shook her head. It was almost as if she had decided that I felt the same way as she did about the girl. I felt sorry for the girl and wanted to intervene. I didn't step in because I felt that it might jeopardise my chances of sorting out the problem I was there for.
>
> I sat in my car in the surgery car park for quite some time after berating myself for not sticking up for the girl. I have wondered since what sort of

effect that dreadful encounter might have had on her, and if it would have any bearing on her visiting the surgery in the future.

Alan, 50-year-old company director

We have all heard stories of how people have not been spoken to in the best way by receptionists on the phone or face-to-face. These unpleasant experiences risk placing patients in a worse state than they were before they made contact. The last thing a doctor wants is a more agitated patient whom he or she is about to consult next. In the case of Alan's story, the receptionist had adopted a high level of status, which moved the young girl into a lower status level where she felt intimidated.

There are many possible reasons why the girl was struggling to express herself clearly. It may have been related to a medical condition or she may have just felt very anxious or self-conscious about visiting the surgery. Regardless of why, this girl needed to feel more comfortable and at ease to explain what she wanted. A mid-level status could have created an atmosphere in which the girl felt more able to do so. The girl needed reassurance from the receptionist that she would do her best to help her.

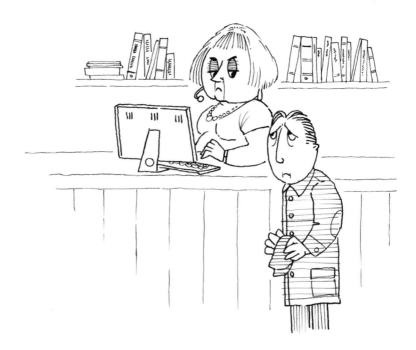

# Physical status

## Story 3: Making judgements on what we see

*Things are not always what they seem; the
first appearance deceives many.*

Ovid

When we meet someone for the first time we make a judgement on what we see. An opinion is being formed, often before any eye contact has been made or there is any vocal interaction. It might be the wrong one, but consciously or subconsciously a view has been taken. It is, therefore, critical that we send out open and neutral physical signals. We do not want to close ourselves off or appear inaccessible. Nigel recalls a memorable patient who demonstrates his concerns by playing high status to the doctor.

It was the most extraordinary experience. A man came to see me complaining of abdominal pain. He was a tall man in his mid-thirties who looked like he kept himself fit. In fact, he appeared rather proud of his physique. After examining him, I felt that his pain was probably muscular and that he might be overdoing things at the gym. He bristled at the suggestion. He sat back in the chair and put his hands behind his head and laughed. Whilst I tried to explain my reasoning, he suddenly stood up. Towering over me, he raised his voice and told me in no uncertain terms that I was wrong and challenged what I knew about training in the gym. I calmly asked him to sit down, so we could talk more about the problem. After a few seconds he sat down in a similar way to which he sat before.

As I explored more what he was worried about, his whole demeanour changed. He started to lean forward with his hands between his legs and spoke in a much softer tone. He appeared more vulnerable and wanted further reassurance that there was nothing seriously wrong. He seemed grateful as he left. I felt relieved it had been resolved amicably. At one point I really did think he wanted to hit me.

Nigel, GP

Worry can cause people to behave in a way that they would not normally. What is interesting is how Nigel handled the situation. He countered a high intimidating physical status with a calm and caring mid-level status. If he had tackled high status with high status, an ugly scene may have ensued. Nigel stayed in control and was able to put the man in a better emotional place than he had been in when they first met.

Of course, doctors can use a high physical status too, but not, one would hope, in such an intimidating and aggressive way. Leaning back in the chair with the head in a reclined position might give us a feeling of confidence but what is it saying to the person we are communicating with? It could be interpreted as overconfidence, arrogance and disinterest, or as feeling superior and dismissive. It may make the patient feel that he or she is being looked down on or merely being tolerated.

The reverse, a low physical status, would be a closed posture that would indicate a physical boundary to our space. It might be saying 'please don't notice me – I'm not actually here'. Overly leaning forward to show interest could be conceived as a weak physicality, which may generate a feeling in the patient of a lack of confidence in the person conducting the consultation.

Folded arms can also send out negative signals from both sides of the status spectrum. They can be a barrier that says: 'I'm not interested in you'. Put a slight tilt of the head with folded arms and you could have: 'I don't believe you'. Folded arms invariably send out a message of some sort and it is usually the wrong sort.

The most confidence-inspiring, non-threatening and comfortable posture for a patient to encounter is the neutral open one – **not** leaning back looking down the nose, **not** leaning forward or being closed off but instead sitting comfortably in the middle of these extremes.

A mid-level physical status is one that is approachable, strong and reassuring. It sends out signals of accessibility and interest, and it allows people to connect.

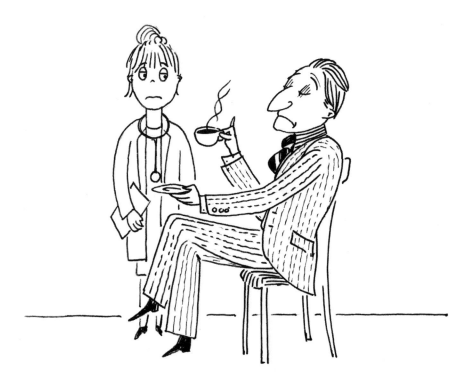

# Vocal status

## Story 4: It's not what you say, it's the way that you say it

What kind of voice do you have? Why are some voices much easier to listen to than others? What we say may be very important but so is how we say it. Our vocal image affects the way our listeners perceive us. A story can be told in many different ways using exactly the same words but differences in vocal delivery will produce contrasting interpretations and meanings. Pitch, tone, pace and volume are all part of vocal delivery, which needs our attention when consulting. The way that Toby's GP spoke to him during a very dramatic incident in his childhood is still as vivid today as it was back then.

> Many years ago when my brother and I were in our teens we became very concerned about Mum. It was the school holidays and Dad was at work. Mum seemed to be drifting in and out of consciousness. She wasn't sleeping. It was the middle of the day and she would never sleep during the day. We called the doctor. By the time he arrived, Mum was not moving at all. She lay rigid with her eyes open, not making a sound. We were in an absolute panic because we thought she was dead. I remember how brilliantly the doctor took control of the situation and calmed us down. He assured us that she was not dead and would be taken to hospital and looked after properly. I can't even remember what he looked like, but I can still recall his words and the way he spoke to us. He seemed so calm and confident that we immediately felt better. Not only did he take care of Mum but he took care of us too.
>
> Toby, 49-year-old software designer

This story demonstrates the power of delivering a message in a tone appropriate to the situation. By using a mid-level of vocal status, calm and confident, the doctor was able to help Toby and his brother regain composure. The same words used with a high vocal status may have caused the boys to feel more agitated. Conversely, the same words spoken with a low vocal status may not have given them the confidence in the doctor that they desperately needed at that time.

The right vocal status makes us accessible. The right vocal status will mirror everything that is good about the right level of physical status. Getting our vocal status right will help our patients to feel able to communicate openly and honestly with us.

Let us explore pitch, tone, pace and volume further.

> *Lord, what an organ is human speech when it is played by a master!*
> Mark Twain

## Pitch

Everyone's voice is unique. Some people speak in a higher register, while others speak much lower. We should be aiming for somewhere in the middle of our natural pitch range. We only need to go two or three notes either side of our natural pitch to create a more interesting vocal delivery.

There have been many people who have tried to change the pitch of their voice, usually by lowering it, to make themselves sound more appealing or authoritative. Margaret Thatcher did this before she became Britain's prime minister, which prompted author and playwright Keith Waterhouse to remark that she always sounded as if she was talking to someone whose dog had just died. Doctors do not want to sound like they lack authority when speaking about medical matters, but equally they do not want to come across as patronising or condescending. It is better to stick with your natural pitch and vary it for interest.

## Tone

> *The art of making deep sounds from the stomach*
> *sound like important messages from the brain.*
> Winston Churchill

Tone is about resonance and intention. The tones we speak with are chosen to have an effect on those we are talking to. When our parents snapped at us 'Don't take that tone of voice with me!' we clearly had upset them, which is probably what we intended to do at the time.

People who use extremes of vocal status tend to have tones that irritate us. The timid whiny tones of the low vocal status and the harsh tones of the high vocal status grate on the ears and make us unwilling listeners. This is why it is important that we listen to ourselves and be selective about the tones we use for different situations. The mid-level warm tones we use within our natural pitch will be the most engaging.

## Pace

Pace relates to how fast or slowly we speak. This is often related to the speed we think and process information, and so part of our personality. If we speak too slowly people may struggle to keep their attention or even feel that they are being patronised. If we speak too quickly there is a risk that our listeners will feel overwhelmed and switch off. Doctors are usually more at risk of talking too quickly, as they attempt to convey significant amounts of information to their patients within relatively short periods of time.

Mid-level vocal speed is the most effective.

## Volume

*He has occasional flashes of silence that make*
*his conversation perfectly delightful.*

The Reverend Sydney Smith

Just as we can be too fast or too slow, we can also be too quiet or too loud. A vocal delivery that is too quiet demonstrates low vocal status and risks our listeners having little confidence in what is said. High volume is associated with a high vocal status, which may be intimidating or overbearing and which risks any information being lost as our listeners move out of a receptive state.

We should aim for mid-level volume every time.

# Emotional status

## Story 5: Empathy and understanding

Our patients experience a wide array of emotions, including feeling anxious, afraid, vulnerable, angry, guilty, depressed, happy, relieved or elated. That is quite some emotional spectrum, and doctors are exposed to this on a daily basis. Emotional status is about how well equipped we are to deal with and manage the feelings of others. Demonstrating empathy and an intuitive understanding of people's needs are essential components. This is what happened when Jim visited his GP soon after his wife had died.

> It was a very difficult time for me. It was only 6 weeks since Louise had died and I wasn't coping too well. Our two girls, both in their mid-teens, were probably handling the situation better than I was. In fact, it was the girls who insisted I went to see the doctor. My doctor couldn't have been more helpful. She listened. I broke down. When she spoke, it was the voice of someone who cared. She had clearly taken in everything I had said. She could so easily have sounded patronising. She spoke quite plainly but with warmth. She looked me in the eye and I could see that she was genuinely concerned for me. She asked about my immediate family and how they were coping. When I left she shook my hand and said that she was here for me if I needed her.
>
> Jim, 56-year-old store manager

This is a moving story about loss and vulnerability. The GP handled this encounter with warmth and sensitivity. She listened and wasn't afraid to look Jim in the eye and let him see that she cared. She asked about the people close to him and at the end of the consultation let him know that he could always contact her again if he needed to.

If we think about the people we are drawn to, they are usually the ones in touch with and in control of their emotions. They are invariably people who appear to be genuinely interested in us, who listen well and make us feel good. These are social abilities that Daniel Goleman describes in his book *Emotional Intelligence* and which 'allow one to shape an encounter, to mobilise and inspire others, to thrive in intimate relationships, to persuade and influence, to put others at ease.'[1]

Successful salespeople take on board a great volume of personal information about their clients and use that information to engage with them. As a result, their clients feel valued and understood and are more likely to do business with them. If doctors are able to do the same, it will help them to manage their patients more effectively and holistically. It is about a personal touch, and we all respond more positively to someone who takes a genuine interest in us.

# Key points

Status is the first 'S' in our model. The level of status we choose in our consultations will affect how we interact with our patients and how they perceive us and interact with us. This is relevant to all staff and colleagues who have patient contact. An open and neutral mid-level status is usually most effective.

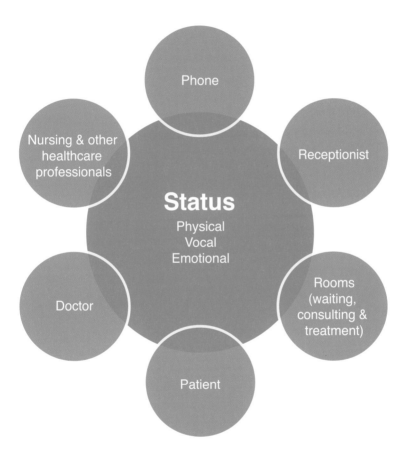

# COMMUNICATION EXERCISE: practising Status

## Physical check

Most consultations will take place sitting down but it is still important to check that we are in a neutral mid-level physical status.

*Do*

✔ Sit straight but relaxed
✔ Shoulders relaxed and square
✔ Legs relaxed, not crossed
✔ Head square on shoulders
✔ Arms and hands relaxed, possibly with hands clasped on lap

*Don't*

✗ Slump back in chair
✗ Lean forwards in chair
✗ Tilt head backwards or to one side
✗ Cross legs
✗ Fold arms

*Expression*

● Neutral but interested
● Good to smile on greeting

*Gestures*

● Few, small and simple

## Emotional check

It is important that we do not carry any extreme emotion into our consultations.

✔ Be aware of any residual emotion carried over from earlier consultations.
✔ Aim for a calm and neutral emotional state (*see* Chapter 6: Sanity for further tips).

## Vocal exercises

Doctors use their voices throughout the day and often have to give presentations. It is important to take care of our voice and make sure that our voice is warmed up and that we have clarity and dexterity of speech. Here are a few quick and simple exercises to keep the voice and speech in good shape.

✔ Gentle humming on one note in the middle of your range

✔ Gentle humming through your whole range

✔ Humming and opening mouth to an 'ah' sound

✔ Humming and opening mouth through each vowel sound

## Group Status exercise

This is a fun exercise you can do very easily with a few colleagues.

Take a pack of playing cards. Remove and put aside the picture cards and jokers. Each of you then takes one of the remaining cards. Do not show your card to the other players. In turn, each player must stand in front of the others and say three things:

1. who he or she is

2. where he or she comes from

3. what he or she does.

These three things must be said in the status level denoted by the number on the card. Ace counts as 1.

1 = Low status (timid and shy)

10 = High status (aloof and arrogant)

The other players must then guess which level of status was being played.

# 2
# Story

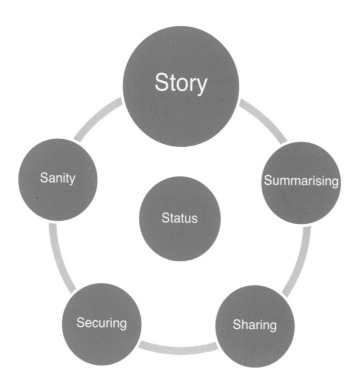

*There have been great societies that did not use the wheel,*
*but there have been no societies that did not tell stories.*

Ursula K Le Guin

*I cannot tell how the truth may be; I say the tale as it was said to me.*

Sir Walter Scott

## What is Story?

Story is defined as a piece of narrative, tale of any length, told or printed in prose or verse, based on either true or fictitious events, legend, myth or anecdote and designed to interest, amuse or instruct the hearer or reader.

Story is the foundation to effective communication. It is how we connect and make sense of our reality. Throughout the ages, great theories, concepts and discoveries have been communicated through story. Outside the world of theatre, there is possibly no other profession as widely touched by the power of story than medicine. Consultation, diagnosis, prevention and cure are all reliant on listening to, digesting, understanding and responding to story. Story is the lifeblood of communication, and the journey that a patient takes us on with his or her story is one of enlightenment.

In this chapter, we will **examine the importance of understanding the patient's story and highlight various factors that may facilitate or impede its telling.**

# Story 1: Making the connection

For many people who seek medical advice, it will be the first time they have met or spoken to a particular doctor. This can be an awkward and unsettling experience for our patients. Making a proper connection is essential if we are going to allow our patients to feel comfortable to tell their story. Here is what happened when Anna called her surgery to speak to her GP about her depression.

> I suffer from intermittent bouts of depression and try as much as I can not to rely on antidepressants. In this particular instance I felt that I could not cope on my own and needed to make an appointment with my GP immediately and get medication. I also felt that I needed to explain how I was feeling and why I needed to see someone straight away. When I called the practice it wasn't possible for me to speak to my usual GP and I was put through to a doctor I did not know. I began to tell the doctor how I was feeling when he interrupted me to ask if I was suicidal. I told him that I wasn't but asked if I could see someone urgently. He told me to hang up, call back the reception and make an appointment in the usual manner. That was the end of our conversation. I felt devastated. I felt that he had not listened to me at all. I felt vulnerable. He had, not in so many words, told me to pull myself together and not waste his time. His lack of interest in what I had to say and his abrupt tone actually made me feel worse than ever.
>
> Anna, 42-year-old auditor

This is an unusual and extreme example of a lack of connection. Most patients appreciate that GPs do not have long periods of time to spend giving advice over the telephone, especially at times when there are people in their waiting rooms needing to be seen. It was unfortunate that Anna called at a time when she could not talk to her own GP, who would have been familiar with her history and with her as a person. The doctor she did speak to did not allow a connection to happen and consequently did not give Anna an opportunity to let him know how serious she felt her condition was. Patients need to feel that they have been 'let in'. This is only possible if the doctor has made him- or herself accessible. A few more considered questions might have put her in a better place emotionally. This can only happen when we allow the patient to connect.

# Story 2: The golden first minute

Can you remember the last time you needed to consult a doctor? Can you remember sitting in the waiting room, clarifying your story in your mind and deciding what you felt you needed to say? George shares some advice from his trainer, about how important that first minute or so is during each consultation.

> My trainer calls it the 'golden first minute'. He believes that most of a patient's story can be elicited during this initial part of the consultation, but only if you allow it. It can be very tempting to get stuck in with more focused questioning about their main complaint, which is what we are taught to do during our hospital training. It wasn't until I started looking back at recorded consultations from my surgeries that I noticed how frequently I interrupted my patients during this initial stage. As a result, I'm sure I missed vital clues and relevant information which would have helped me manage these cases better. I think I was too aware of the limited time I had with each patient and was worried they would talk and talk if I didn't intervene. I realise now, that most patients have said what they wanted to say in the first 30 seconds!
>
> George, GP trainee

Most patients have rehearsed what they want to say to their doctor before they are seen. They want to share their story with the doctor in the hope that they will understand their concerns and be able to help. As George has discovered early on in his general practice training, it can be all too easy to interrupt the patient's initial flow with your own medical agenda.

A useful starting point to consider with all patients you see is 'what has brought them to see me *today*?' What factors have caused them sufficient concern to seek my opinion? What are they hoping I will be able to do for them? Most of this information should be accessible from the patient within the first minute or two, if handled skilfully. Using **open questioning**, which seeks more descriptive replies, is more likely to achieve this. Examples of open questions may include:

*'Tell me more about . . .'*
*'What do you think may be causing . . .?'*
*'You seem very upset by this. What impact has this had on . . .?'*

The use of more closed questioning has its role too, but usually after the patient's agenda has been identified. Closed questions typically result in more specific responses and are useful when clarifying diagnoses and excluding red flag symptoms.

## Story 3: I am listening

A crucial component of story and storytelling is the ability to listen properly to other people's stories. Simply hearing is not enough. We have to listen. Listening involves us giving our complete attention to what we are being told and taking notice of, acting on and responding to what someone has said. When we do listen, and not just hear, we put ourselves into a very strong position to be effective communicators, problem solvers, diagnosticians and healers. Here is a story – someone's account of being listened to.

> It struck me so forcibly that I shall never forget him. He had qualities which I had never seen in any other man. Never had I seen such concentrated attention. There was none of the piercing 'soul penetrating gaze' business. His eyes were mild and gentle. His voice was low and kind. His gestures were few. But the attention he gave me, his appreciation of what I said, even when I said it badly, was extraordinary. You have no idea what it meant to be listened to like that.
>
> A man describing a consultation with Sigmund Freud

This story is taken from Dale Carnegie's book *How to Win Friends and Influence People*,[2] a book that was written in 1936 and which has sold over 16 million copies worldwide. One of the principal themes in Carnegie's book is listening – listening and hearing. He talks of understanding and putting ourselves in someone else's shoes and seeing things from their perspective. The right kind of listening is essential to great communication in consultation.

**Active listening** is what we need to be doing. Listening with genuine interest to every word. Giving our undivided attention. Not looking at a computer screen when someone is speaking. Showing that we understand and respect the opinions of others. We explore this in more depth in Chapter 3: Summarising.

The following are some different types of listening to look out for and avoid.

- **Arrogant listening**: we will all have suffered at the hands of the arrogant listener at some stage of our lives. This is the sort of listener who responds to what is being said with a 'yeah, yeah, I knew that already and I know more than you anyway' kind of attitude. Arrogant listeners are not listening properly or effectively.

- **Selective listening**: this is listening for particular things and ignoring anything else. Selective listeners only hear what they want to hear.
- **Interrupted listening**: this is when the listener does not always let people finish what they are saying and may even finish people's sentences for them as if the listener has made up his or her mind how the story ends. Such listeners are not allowing the proper information to arrive because they are not in fact listening.
- **Aggressive listening**: aggressive listeners are so busy using exaggerated body language and expression to demonstrate how earnestly they are listening, they are at risk of not hearing exactly what is being said.
- **Partial listening**: the partial listener may have good intentions towards the person they are interacting with but becomes distracted. The distraction can be caused by internal thoughts or by something that the other person has said, but by the time proper listening has resumed, the thread of the conversation may have been lost.

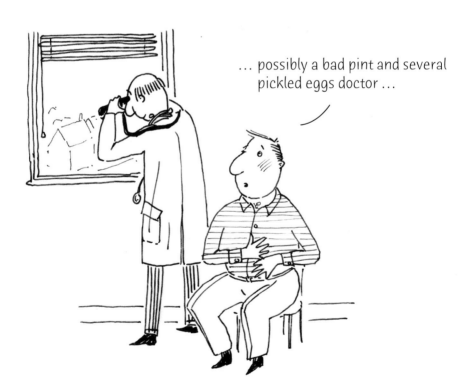

# Story 4: What are you really worried about?

Quite often, our patients do not give their full story and it becomes the doctor's job to find out what is really being said. In Richard's story, one of his patients has a relatively minor complaint. However, underlying this is a far more serious worry that has been troubling him.

> A man I knew reasonably well joined me in the consulting room. He was by no means a frequent visitor to the surgery, in fact this was the first occasion I had seen him there. Our children went to the same school and we had chatted many times in the past at school functions and dropping off the children. After a brief chat about the children and our spouses I asked how I could help. He said that he had a sore throat. His throat was a little red but no white spots. I asked him whether that was all or was there anything else making him feel unwell? He said that there wasn't and I gave some suggestions of how to take care of his throat without using antibiotics, as I didn't think it was that serious. We chatted a little more about families and he didn't seem to be in any hurry to leave. I began to feel that there was something he wasn't telling me, so I asked if there was anything he was worried about. It turned out that he had recently spent some time with an old friend who had since developed meningitis and the first symptom was a sore throat.
>
> Richard, GP

Stories very often have subplots and their characters may say one thing when the subtext tells us something different. This was clearly the case with Richard's patient. Richard's senses told him something was wrong. A young, healthy man he only sees at school events turns up at his surgery with a sore throat? He then stays on for more idle chit-chat? A little reading between the lines of the innocent story unearths the real reason for the visit. The man probably felt rather silly going to the surgery for a consultation rather than to the pharmacist for some lozenges, but there was a very real concern that he might have something life-threatening.

Patient health beliefs are not always easy to dig out. Unless we actively seek to explore these, we may not truly identify what our patients are concerned about and what they may be expecting from their doctor. Unidentified health beliefs may manifest themselves in an awkwardness or embarrassment when talking about why they are there. Or they may present with something simple or trivial, as was the case with Richard's patient. Doctors must always be ready to identify a story's subplot and understand the importance of eliciting the vital subtext that will lead them to what the patient may not be telling them.

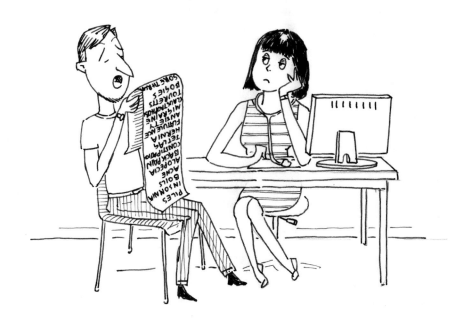

# Story 5: Cultural differences

Why is it that some patients are much easier to connect with than others? How aware and sensitive are you to each of your patient's traditions, values, beliefs and behaviours, especially if they differ from your own? Different groups of people have different stories to tell, and they tell them in different ways. Heidi describes an interesting encounter with a patient who, perhaps because of her cultural background, found it hard to tell hers.

> A young woman of Indian origin came to see me. I greeted her in what I like to think is my usual warm manner and invited her to sit down. She seemed uncomfortable with our situation from the beginning. There was barely any eye contact and, because of the way she mumbled, it was difficult to understand what she was saying. I gathered from the little I did understand that her English, although quite good, was that of someone who had not been in the country for very long. Which made me wonder why she did not have anyone with her to help with the consultation. I tried to clarify several times what it was she had attended for, but each time she could not look at me and found it difficult to say anything at all.
>
> I asked if she had specifically requested to see a female doctor. She said, 'yes'. I then asked if it was to do with a 'woman's health issue'. She said, 'yes'. I continued to ask questions hoping one would lead me to the root of her problem, if indeed there was one. This went on for some considerable time, and I began to think of the room of patients outside waiting to see me. I admit I became rather frustrated and a little irritated with her, which must have shown when I finally said, 'I really can't help you, if you don't tell me!' She stood up to leave but somehow I managed to get her to sit down again. After another long pause, it suddenly occurred to me that there was one obvious question I had not asked yet. 'Are you in a sexual relationship?' She hung her head and did not answer. My next question hit the spot faster than all the others. 'Would you like some form of contraception?' She looked up, her eyes full of tears, and nodded.
>
> Heidi, GP

There are so many different cultures in the world and it is this diversity that can make a doctor's job both fascinating and challenging. Doctors, more than most, rely on heightened sensitivity and intuition to operate on a daily basis. Each patient will have a unique set of personal characteristics, shaped by his or her past experiences. Family, friends, society, religious and spiritual influences can play a significant part in the way we perceive ourselves and others and, ultimately, how we communicate with one another.

Heidi's story is an intriguing one that raises many questions. It is likely we will all have our own opinion as to why this consultation was so awkward. Whether our reasons differ or not may reflect the fact that we, as doctors, are also individually different too. Heidi certainly had mixed feelings about the way she handled this particular consultation. Was she the best choice of GP for this young woman? Would it have been better for her to have seen a female doctor from the same ethnic background? How would she have coped seeing a male doctor? Will she come back again to see Heidi?

Developing an awareness of how differently individual patients communicate their needs and concerns is essential for successful consultation. Intercultural competence is an area of training that major global businesses are beginning to invest in, to ensure their organisations are applying the necessary skills to be as productive and profitable as they can. Valuing Diversity training already exists within most general practice training schemes, but is it sufficient for today's modern society? With the increasing desire for intercultural competence, perhaps it falls upon the medical profession to lead the way in promoting a greater awareness and understanding of this challenging area?

## Story 6: A story shared

I recently needed to talk to a doctor about increasing my medication but was unable to see my GP, as she was away that day. Instead I saw a very warm friendly young lady who listened attentively to everything I said. She seemed very understanding of my problems and didn't hurry me, although I knew that my appointment was for 10 minutes only. She was a new doctor to the practice, born in another country, and as I am interested in people I asked her about her life whilst she was writing my prescription. In less than a couple of minutes she was able to give me a few interesting facts about herself. When I got up to leave and held out my hand, she rose from her chair and put both of her hands around mine. I felt special and valued, and that we had in some way bonded.

Christine, 78-year-old retired receptionist

It is interesting that Christine felt that this experience had brought about a bonding. It really doesn't take very much to let a short story create a feeling of warmth and friendliness. This is a sweet story about a brief sharing of stories that is a convenient prelude to our last story in this chapter.

# Story 7: Doctor who?

What's your story? How well do you know yourself? How would your friends or family describe you? What life experiences, above and beyond your basic medical training, do you bring to your role as a doctor? How would your patients describe you? In our final story of this chapter we look at the relationship that Story has with Status. This is what happened when Marcus met one of his patients outside surgery hours.

> It was a warm Sunday morning and there was an open-air market in the town where we live. My wife and I decided to take our two young children to the market, where they could have fun on the bouncy castle and the other amusements laid on for the kids while we explored what was on offer at the stalls. We had only just arrived when we were approached by one of my patients who was with a couple of her friends. She seemed really eager to introduce me to her friends who, as far as I was aware, were not patients of the practice. She was so effusive in her praise of me it was rather embarrassing, telling her friends that I was the best doctor in the area, with the best colleagues and the best surgery. I tried to deflect attention from myself by introducing her to my wife and children but she went on. She told my wife what a lucky woman she was to have me and she told my children how proud they must be to have such a lovely and clever Daddy, and on and on it went! Eventually we managed to extricate ourselves. My wife looked at me and said cheekily 'do you have this effect on all your female patients?!'
>
> Marcus, GP

The influence of the doctor's story can be a powerful one. A doctor's story is also their brand. Jeff Bezos, the founder of Amazon, said 'Your brand is what people say about you when you are not in the room'. Marcus' brand seems to be held in high regard by the person he met at the market. But not all doctors will be perceived in the same way, and not all patients will feel the same way about the same doctor.

Our story and our brand have a very strong link to status. There is a high positional status that doctors have within a community and it is important that the perceived status is supporting it well. We all need to take a deep look at our own story and how it constitutes our perceived brand, and whether this best represents the bigger brand of our practice. There are many factors that may influence our patients and their decision to seek our opinion. Some we have little choice over, such as age, gender and natural appearance. However, there are other factors we may have more control over, such as known previous experience, additional expertise, reputation, how well you run to time, and how well you listen, to name but a few.

It is worth mentioning 'burnout' here. Doctors work in high-pressure environments and are exposed to much suffering and death. There is a risk of becoming mechanical, detached and emotionally blunted. Part of burnout is a sense of depersonalisation. We disconnect from our own story. If we disconnect from our own story, it is more likely we will disconnect from our patients' stories too. Which is why keeping our sanity is so important, as we will explore later in this book.

We should constantly be asking questions about ourselves. What do I feel strongly about? What are my aims? What are my goals? What are my values? Do I care what people think of me? We should care. The way patients feel about us may influence their story and how they tell it. This is where feedback from patients and colleagues can help give you a more objective viewpoint.

# Key points

Story is the second 'S' in our model. It is at the very heart of the human condition, which is why it is especially important in the medical world. It allows us to connect with those we are trying to help. We must listen properly to the patient's story. We need to be sensitive to any diverse backgrounds that may influence the story we are listening to. We have to listen out for the unheard and interpret the subtext. We need to be aware of how we are being perceived through our own story.

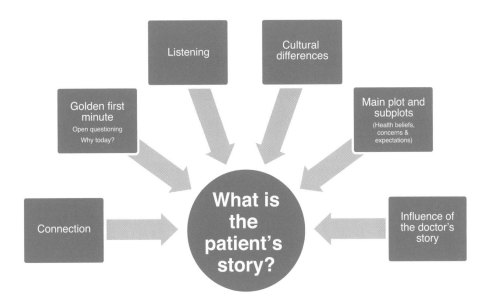

---

### COMMUNICATION EXERCISE: practising Story

Here is a useful exercise that you can practise with your colleagues.

- In pairs, tell a colleague the story of a particular case that you found interesting, using only the salient points that brought you to your diagnosis. Try not to let this story run for more than 1 minute.
- Tell the story again, but this time take 5 minutes and bring in other outside influences that might have had an influence on your diagnosis, such as other people in the story, feelings, perceptions and personal background.

Swap roles and repeat.

---

**Consider**: instead of asking 'what's the problem?' perhaps we should be asking 'what's the story?'

# 3

# Summarising

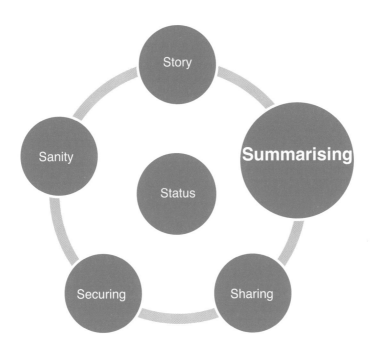

*If you want to know how I feel, I'll summarise it in one word – terrible!*

Gary Bettman

*To summarize: it is a well-known fact that those people who most want to rule people are, ipso facto, those least suited to do it. To summarize the summary: anyone who is capable of getting themselves made President should on no account be allowed to do the job. To summarize the summary of the summary: people are a problem.*

Douglas Adams

# What is Summarising?

Summarising is defined as 'making a summary'. It is a process of reviewing what has been said and done during a conversation, and of providing a succinct résumé of the essential points. Its purpose is not to explain, judge or interpret, but to review understanding.

Summarising will enhance your encounters with patients, their families and your colleagues. It is by no means a new concept and we recognise that others such as Roger Neighbour (*The Inner Consultation*) have appreciated its importance.[3] It is widely recognised as an essential tool in the business world. Try searching the Internet – you will find a whole array of communication skills training courses that focus on just this. Yet, it is a step in our communication process that is frequently overlooked.

There are many different introductory phrases that one can use to start the summarising process, such as:

> *'So, what you are saying is . . .'*
> *'From what you have just told me, my understanding is . . .'*
> *'Can I check that I've heard/understood you correctly . . .?'*

These will undoubtedly be modified according to the situation. We do not offer any prescriptive tips, but we suggest that as well as checking your understanding is correct, your summary remains neutral, without blame or your personal judgement, and that it is concise, with relevant and important information only. It should not include your opinion or what you think the patient should have said. It needs to reflect as true an account as possible of what the patient is thinking and feeling.

After reading this chapter, we believe you will have a better understanding of **what summarising is, how it will help you and others you communicate with, and how you can learn to summarise more effectively**.

# Story 1: 'Did the doc hear all that I said?'

How do you know if you've been listened to? How can you tell if the person you are talking to has properly understood what you are saying? Our next story comes from Chris, who is struggling generally, both at work and home, because of high levels of stress and anxiety.

> I was experiencing a lot of stress at work. My manager was struggling too and it was beginning to affect my home life. I wasn't sleeping or eating properly and I was becoming increasingly irritable around my wife and children. It was when I started to develop a whole array of strange physical symptoms such as pins and needles in both my hands that I decided to seek the advice of my doctor. I had worked myself up into a bit of a tiz. You read stories about how stress can make you ill, and I really thought my body was 'falling apart'. The doctor greeted me warmly, listened to what I had to say and then suggested that I was suffering with severe anxiety. At the end of the consultation, I left with a prescription for some pills to try and a follow-up appointment in 3 weeks. I'm not sure I was reassured at the time that all my physical symptoms were attributable to my stress and anxiety. To be honest, I don't know if the doctor actually took in all my various complaints. I know they only have 10 minutes per person and I did have a lot to say.
>
> Chris, 32-year-old office worker

Stress and anxiety are common complaints. They present real challenges to the GP, both diagnostically and with time management. From a medical viewpoint, it would appear that the GP in this story did well to manage the volume of information provided by Chris and come up with an acceptable plan of action and follow-up. Yet, Chris is not entirely satisfied with the encounter. He is not sure the doctor heard his full story properly. Why is this? What would have reassured Chris that all his 'various complaints' had been noted?

Let us assume that the doctor did hear and took on board all of Chris' concerns. The challenge, then, was communicating this back to the patient. We feel this story highlights a need for doctors to **acknowledge** what patients have been saying. Doctors may listen and offer advice, but most people initially seek an acknowledgement of their symptoms, feelings, worries and responses. We would go further and say a **non-judgemental** acknowledgement. Acknowledgement is a powerful tool and strategy, and one that breeds trust and openness.

Perhaps if the doctor had summarised the story well, Chris would have felt more reassured that all his points had been 'taken on board'. There are obvious emotional advantages for the patient. They are more likely to feel they have been listened to and taken seriously, which in turn improves rapport. It reflects a doctor who is interested and wants to understand.

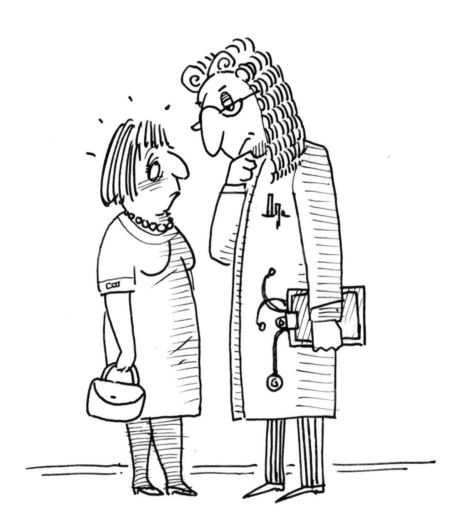

# Story 2: 'I want antibiotics – the last doctor missed my tonsillitis!'

This case involves a patient who makes a complaint about the previous management of his sore throat. He has a recurrence of this problem but this time is quite firm with the doctor about what he thinks he needs. How can these differences be reconciled?

> I was having a joint surgery with my trainer. It's a common situation – people often come in asking for antibiotics for their coughs and sore throats. I end up spending ages with them, explaining the differences between bacteria and viruses, as well as the current evidence for antibiotics. Well, our next patient came in expecting just that, for a 3-day sore throat. He also complained that another doctor in the practice had missed his tonsillitis only a couple of months ago, and as a result he endured almost a week of pain and misery!
>
> My trainer was in the 'hot seat' this time. I was amazed how calm she was throughout and how effective she was in dealing with this patient. The patient left the room with only advice (no prescription!) and said 'thank you' on his way out!
>
> My epiphany was recognising how engaged the patient became during my trainer's initial summary. As she summarised this patient's story, concerns and health beliefs, the patient was nodding and saying 'yes'. She had the patient already agreeing with her before they had even started discussing management issues. I had not considered how effective a technique this had been.
>
> Charlie, GP trainee

When summarising includes a complaint, it becomes even more important that we demonstrate we have heard and understood correctly what has been said. We do not have to agree with the patient's viewpoint or even feel that what has been said is true. Our aim is to acknowledge rather than validate and, by doing so, open up the channels that will enable our patients to listen to us when we go on to express our opinions.

Is this not the case in most conversations? How do you feel when you are talking to someone who is more interested in what he or she has to say than what you say? Start to lose interest? Stop listening? Many self-help books have been written since Dale Carnegie's worldwide success of *How to Win Friends and Influence People* (1936), and being a good listener crops up time and time again as one of the top factors in being an effective communicator. Summarising demonstrates to your patient that you have been just that, a good listener.

It is more challenging where there is a potential conflict of views. We want to defuse any negative emotions, and avoid defensive behaviours that are likely to stifle the flow of our consultations. Finding common ground will enable both patient and doctor to work together towards agreed results. Charlie, the GP trainee, has first-hand experience of how effective summarising can be in facilitating this process.

# Story 3: A sudden realisation

Many consultations involve third parties, such as carers, family or friends. Jane has come along to support her mother. Both come away with more than they had expected.

> My elderly mother is fiercely independent, despite a multitude of physical problems. Her mind, though, is as sharp as a tack! She loves her GP and thinks she's wonderful. I've accompanied my mum on a couple of occasions, and found her doctor to be very approachable and chatty. It must be a real challenge for the doctor to deal with all my mother's ongoing complaints. However, it wasn't until we saw one of the other doctors in the practice (her usual GP was on holiday) that I got a true sense of what was going on with my mum's health and how rapidly she was declining. Perhaps it was because he had not seen my mum before, but he went through all her various complaints over the previous months to date, and I suppose helped my mum and me to see things more objectively. It suddenly became obvious that we needed to take action now about making changes to my mother's home set-up.
>
> Jane, 67-year-old daughter

Summarising can highlight important or special points. It helps to clarify what has happened and been said. It offers all parties involved in a conversation the opportunity to reflect on their understanding of that particular situation. With patients who are well known to you, it can be easy to make assumptions. In this scenario, it is likely that the new doctor was summarising the story to help him (rather than the patient) understand the complexity of the case. Yet by doing so, he enabled both Jane and her mother to gain additional insights into her declining health.

This encounter occurred face-to-face. Consider the additional challenges had this taken place over the telephone instead. In the absence of non-verbal cues, clarification becomes crucial. This is particularly pertinent when communicating with third parties, where misunderstandings are more likely to occur. A doctor's duty is ultimately to the patient and it is vital that we place ourselves in a position to gather the salient facts and details to make a proper assessment.

# Story 4: So many problems!

Doctors are often confronted by patients with multiple and complex complaints, both physical and psychological. Sarah, a GP in training, is having a difficult morning at work and encounters one such patient.

> It was awful. I was already running late during my morning surgery. My next patient had only just registered at our practice that day, so we had no previous medical records for her. Before she had even sat down, she burst into tears and then disclosed how terrible she was feeling. She had recently moved into the local area with two young children, her husband had just lost his job, she was experiencing panic attacks, low mood, drank too much alcohol in the evenings and was concerned that her eating disorder from teenage years had come back. I didn't know where to start. I felt overwhelmed with the number of issues she was telling me about. In the end I tried to address each problem individually, but when I did, she started talking about another issue that was causing her distress. I spent at least 40 minutes with her. My other patients waiting to see me were not happy.
>
> Sarah, GP trainee

Even the most skilled and experienced GP would find Sarah's case a challenge. Which point should Sarah address first? How can she manage it all in a single appointment without running late? Summarising may not be the only answer to these questions but what it will allow is a short pause for reflection. Sarah has been hit by a tidal wave of distress and emotion. It is hard not to be overwhelmed by this. In these circumstances, we would argue that summarising becomes even more important. Sarah needs to clarify with herself, as well as her patient, what is going on. This in turn will set up the opportunity for them to prioritise what needs to be addressed today and what can wait.

Although this case highlights the difficulties in dealing with psychological illness, many patients present doctors with their 'lists' of problems. The elderly and those with chronic disease often have more than one issue to discuss. Mastering the skills of acknowledgement and clarification will aid you in your negotiations with the patient as to what can realistically be achieved in the allocated time.

# Story 5: The hidden agenda

Eliciting a patient's worries and fears can be a tricky business. Mental health and issues around sex are areas that most people feel awkward talking about. Certain patients, like teenagers, even more so. Often these issues lie hidden throughout the consultation or are revealed at the end when time is limited. If you want to discover why patients attend when they do, and to advise and reassure them more effectively, then understanding their hidden feelings and fears is essential. Simon's encounter with a worried mum illustrates this.

> I recall one of my first consultations as a new GP partner with a very anxious mum and her toddler. Her child had been coughing for over a week and was a little off his food. Looking through the medical records, mum attended frequently with minor coughs and colds, and I assumed that mum lacked confidence in managing simple self-limiting illness. However, it wasn't until I fed back to mum what I understood she was worried about that she actually admitted to her fear that her son may have cystic fibrosis. I had initially asked her if there was anything specific she was concerned about, but it wasn't until my summary, bringing the whole story together and in context, that the mum felt able to vocalise her biggest fear.
>
> Simon, GP trainer

Opening up our innermost thoughts and feelings can be hard enough to do with those that we love and are most close to. Doctors should not rely on their professional status alone for patients to disclose all the relevant information, which may be very sensitive and intimate. There may be clues in the patient's non-verbal behaviour that a hidden agenda may exist, such as poor eye contact, appearing nervous or seeming embarrassed. Doctors should also be aware of their own hidden agendas that may affect the consultation (e.g. wanting to finish quickly or incentives to reduce referral rates).

What is interesting in Simon's case is that he had asked the anxious mum directly about any specific concerns early on in the consultation, yet she did not feel comfortable to disclose her fear about cystic fibrosis until his summary. This reflects that sometimes we **need to revisit** an issue to allow individuals to open up more. Summarising should be an interactive process, encouraging a mutual trust and respect, thereby allowing individuals to lower their defences and express how they truly feel to their doctor. Useful phrases such as *'Have I covered everything?'* or *'Is there anything else not mentioned yet that is bothering you?'* can help to bring the process of summarising to a close, and give the patient the opportunity to raise anything that they may have felt too uncomfortable to do earlier.

# Story 6: 'It's what makes being a doctor so much fun!'

I've been a GP for 20 years and love it. For me, I particularly enjoy the detective work, trying to decipher the relevant detail from each person's tale. You could say we are the 'Sherlock Holmes' of the medical world. And just as Sherlock gives his dramatic summations after gathering all the evidence, I too believe in the power of summarising the findings, clarifying with the patient that the data I have gathered do indeed match up with his or her own understanding. It may sound like an easy skill to learn, but it has taken me several years to master, and use it I do with often dramatic effect.

John, GP trainer

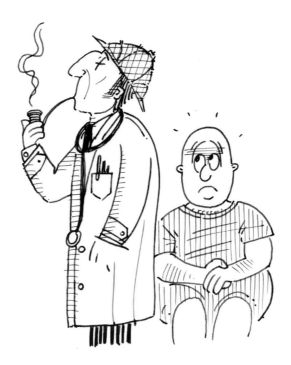

# Key points

Summarising is the third 'S' in our model. It brings together the important features of the patient's 'Story' so far. It allows the patient to feel that they have been listened to and understood through the process of acknowledgement, and enables both the doctor and patient to clarify any relevant points. Later in the consultation, you will be offering your opinion and advice. Making sure that patients feel understood will encourage them to try to understand you.

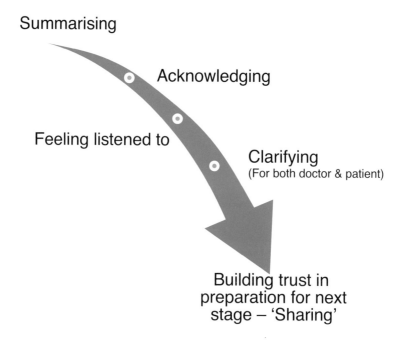

# COMMUNICATION EXERCISE: practising Summarising

Think of an occasion when you were involved with a patient, colleague, family or friend and it didn't go as well as you had hoped and has not been fully resolved. How has this made you feel? What, in your mind, were the main issues? What would you ideally have liked to happen next?

(This exercise requires a minimum of two people, ideally more.)

*Part 1*: Pair up and tell your story to your colleague. Others in the group remain in an observational role, with the opportunity to give feedback later.

*Part 2*: Your colleague must now summarise what he or she has heard and understood. Remember, this is an interactive process and should involve the storyteller.

*Part 3*: The storyteller now feeds back to the summariser how he or she felt during the summarising process.

*Part 4*: Constructive comments from others in the group observing. Were there any key phrases used that worked well? What helped to make the summarising effective? What didn't help? Consider rehearsing any good suggestions for improvement.

Now swap over, with someone else telling his or her story, and another practising his or her summarising skills.

# 4
# Sharing

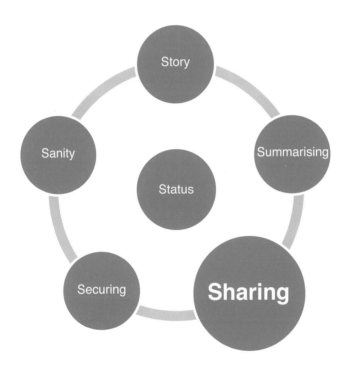

*We confirm our reality by sharing.*

Barbara Harrison

*If you have an apple and I have an apple and we exchange apples, then you and I will still each have one apple. But if you have an idea and I have an idea and we exchange these ideas, then each of us will have two ideas.*

George Bernard Shaw

# What is Sharing?

The word 'communication' comes from the Latin word *communicare*, which means 'to share', and to share is defined as using or doing something jointly. In the context of a medical consultation, sharing involves an interactive exchange of information between the doctor and patient, including individual health beliefs, any concerns or specific expectations. To share, this process must involve both the patient *and* the doctor.

'Sharing' marks a shift of emphasis from data gathering to managing patients' current problems. What seems on the surface a simple and straightforward concept, in reality provides a significant challenge to many doctors, especially those new to general practice. Traditionally, doctors have been used to *giving* their advice to patients or *telling* them what they need to do. This is still very much the case in hospital practice, where doctor-centred consulting remains the norm across most specialties.

So why share? Is this just more modern-day 'touchy-feely' GP psychobabble?

In this chapter we will explain **what 'Sharing' is within a medical consultation, why it is important to both you and your patients, and how you can do it effectively**.

# Story 1: Managing a problem rather than a diagnosis

Our first story comes from Amanda. She reflects on the differences between her hospital and general practice training.

> It was a significant mind shift for me. During my hospital training, the main focus was to exclude disease. So when I started my first GP post, I felt a real pressure and expectation to come up with a specific diagnosis with each patient. Yet, most of the time I couldn't. It felt very uncomfortable. I now realise that much of general practice involves managing our patients' beliefs and concerns, as well as their physical ailments, and this requires a more holistic approach. There needs to be more discussion with the patient, rather than the doctor telling them what to do.
>
> Amanda, newly qualified GP

The vast majority of people seeking medical advice is seen and managed within general practice. Most will not have any serious or significant disease and so managing individual illness behaviour is an important aspect of a GP's role. In hospitals, however, people are seeking to exclude, or requesting help in managing, specific diseases, which may not be possible in the community. Illness and disease are different entities, although there will be frequent overlap. How you choose to approach these with your patients will affect how you manage them.

Amanda's transition into general practice was a struggle as she attempted to move from a 'disease-centred' model of consulting to one more 'patient-' or 'problem-centred'. Knowing what the patient is worried about and his or her opinion as to what may be causing the problem is key to this sharing stage of the consultation. Your opinion may well differ from your patient's. You may have no definitive diagnosis to offer. As Amanda highlights, discussion and sharing of opinions is therefore essential.

# Story 2: A simple case of high cholesterol?

'Prevention is better than cure' is a philosophy held by many in the medical pro-fession. GPs are well placed in the community to promote good health and target certain patient groups opportunistically. Our daily newspapers and magazines are full of articles advising people to do this and try that to keep themselves healthy and to live longer. Yet, often when doctors attempt to advise on such matters, their advice goes unheeded. Why should this be? Louise, a GP trainee, describes her dif-ficulties in persuading one of her patients to take her advice.

> It should have been a straightforward consultation, but it wasn't. This fit and healthy 50-year-old man came to see me following a private medical examination, arranged through his work. It had flagged up a high cho-lesterol reading of almost 10. Everything else was normal. He exercised regularly, his diet seemed healthy and he had a normal body mass index score. So, I advised that he try a statin to bring his cholesterol level down. However, he remained resistant to this, despite my explanations of the risks if left untreated. It was a surprisingly long consultation too, and both of us appeared to be dissatisfied at the end.
>
> It transpired later in the year, that he had actually come back and seen my trainer soon after our encounter. They had agreed to a trial of lifestyle and dietary strategies for 6 months. When a repeat blood test showed just a marginal improvement he opted for the statin. Looking back, I realise now that I had not really shared the options with him. I had been more focused on the high blood test result than my patient's thoughts and feelings about it. My trainer had achieved what I tried to do but had done so by involving the patient more in the decision making.
>
> Louise, GP trainee

The decision to see a doctor is usually an active choice made by patients. They want to tell you their story and find out what your professional opinion is. However, the decision whether to take your advice and subsequently follow any action plan will depend on a number of factors. Perhaps the single most important factor is whether they agree with you. Patient consent means just that – they agree, not forced against their will, and not following your advice blindly either.

Compliance with any treatment or management plan will be influenced by the degree of agreement from the patient. Agreement normally arises from a sharing of minds, an appreciation of any differences and negotiation. Louise was aware of the advice she needed to give medically about raised cholesterol, but she stumbled in her attempt to negotiate her patient's 'wants' into perceived 'needs'. Her trainer succeeded in eliciting this patient's beliefs and incorporating them into a shared plan that was mutually acceptable. The eventual decision to start taking a statin became an active choice by the patient.

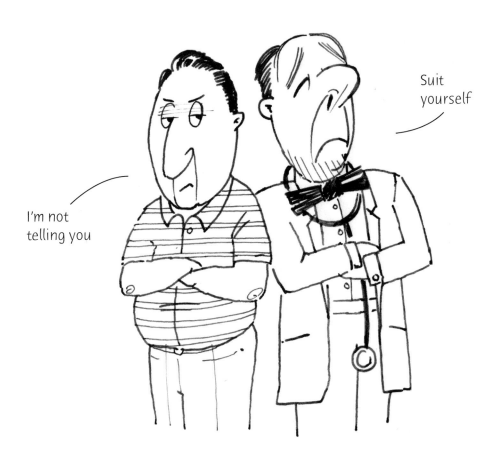

# Story 3: 'I don't know what it is'

How confident are you in dealing with what you don't know? How do you respond to a patient sitting in front of you, hoping for a solution to a problem you don't have? Jill gives her opinion on this matter.

> I think most people expect their doctor to have an answer to what is causing their symptoms. And I think most doctors expect that of themselves. Yet my doctor often shares with me the things he is not certain or sure about. Don't get me wrong, I think he is excellent and he is very popular. It's just that you get an honest and clearer picture of what he is thinking. Somehow, it feels more real, and I come away more reassured, even though we may not know what exactly the problem may be!
>
> Jill, 63-year-old retired teacher

Sharing may also include what you do not know. There are not many things in life we can say with 100% certainty. Most people accept and understand this. Doctors are human too. In the appropriate context, revealing this to our patients can prove therapeutic as well as aiding trust and rapport. We can stand alongside our patients and help them to face their uncertain futures, as much as our own.

You may have come across the joke 'What's the difference between God and a doctor? God knows he's not a doctor!' This reflects a stereotypical and outdated view of the traditional doctor, who pretended to know everything, and their word was bible. Times have changed, as have training, public expectations and increased litigation. Doctors have a responsibility to provide their patients with the relevant information to make an informed decision. By sharing with them what we know, as well as what we are less certain about, we are encouraging our patients to take more ownership of their own care.

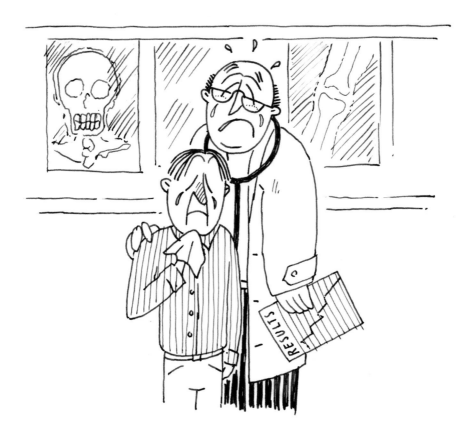

# Story 4: A specialist's viewpoint

In the medical world, is a GP a 'Jack of all trades, but master of none'? Peter, an ear, nose and throat consultant, thinks not and highlights a skill that GPs need to acquire and become expert in – that of managing uncertainty.

> I really do admire GPs. I don't think I've got what it takes to be one. I would struggle with all the 'not knowing'. Literally, anything can come through your door and you can't be an expert in everything. At least in my specialist field, I can tell my patients whether they have a particular disease, structural problem or not. I have the luxury of using a naso-endoscope in clinic to examine the upper aero-digestive tract, or arranging a scan to image specific areas of the head and neck more fully if needed. I like to know things with certainty and reassure my patients likewise.
>
> Peter, ear, nose and throat consultant

A significant challenge for GPs is managing uncertainty. Decisions need to be made without the wider team of doctors and other medical professionals that exist in a hospital environment. Patients have not been pre-assessed by a casualty doctor, or 'worked-up' by a more junior member of the team. Few investigations are immediately accessible to aid diagnosis, and time is limited too. Most of the patients Peter sees are referred to him by other doctors (usually GPs) and with specific questions and requests. The psychosocial aspects of their lives are unlikely to be addressed.

One GP trainee we spoke to described the transition from hospital to general practice as 'akin to walking out onto the battlefield without a sword or a shield'. This is an interesting analogy, reflecting a perceived vulnerability and lack of armoury to manage his or her patient encounters and a significant chasm between two medical worlds. No consultation should ever be a 'battle'. You are the patients' advocate and your biggest asset within your consultations is your patients. Use them. Include them. Share with them.

We need to recognise and accept that uncertainty is an inevitable part of life. Only by doing so can we incorporate this within our consultations, strengthen the decision-making process and help break down any unrealistic expectations that patients and doctors may have of themselves or each other.

# A difference of opinion: a doctor's perspective

## Story 5: 'I want more time off work!'

Our final two stories in this chapter focus on managing conflicting opinions between doctors and patients. What strategies do you use to aid resolution? James reflects on a memorable request for a sick note.

> We had completely different opinions. He felt that more time off work was what he needed. I felt the opposite. It seemed he was disengaging more and more from his workplace, making it harder eventually to return. We were reaching a stalemate. He was becoming increasingly frustrated and thought I was being a barrier to his recovery.
>
> After acknowledging our different viewpoints, I asked him how he felt we could move forward. He initially seemed surprised by this question, as if he had expected my decision to be final, one way or the other. Somehow, his defensive manner changed to one of collaboration. Sharing this responsibility in deciding how best to manage his recovery and 'return to normal life' triggered something within him, which resulted in him being more engaged and proactive. We eventually agreed to a phased return to work over the following month. All parties, including his employer, were happy with this arrangement.
>
> James, GP

Requests for sick notes are common in general practice. Most are straightforward to manage, but there are always a few that pose more of a challenge. There are many reasons why people find returning to work difficult after periods of sickness, especially if related to mental health. Doctors often feel a real conflict within themselves as they try to act in their patients' best interests, promoting their recovery, but at the same time feeling that they are somehow 'policing the state' and discouraging those that may be 'playing the system' or 'needing a gentle push' to get back to work.

In this instance, there is an initial difference between what this patient wants and what the doctor believes he needs. James has negotiated and collaborated well by sharing the responsibility to resolve their current dilemma. Consequently, they were able to work together on an outcome that was mutually acceptable to all involved.

It is not uncommon for people to become agitated during periods of conflict. It is important to remain calm and listen. Let the patient have his or her say. Empathise and acknowledge what he or she has said and then appeal to that individual to hear your views. Be clear why you do not agree with his or her views and explain what you are happy to do instead. If possible, try to end on a positive note – is there a win–win solution?

# A difference of opinion: a patient's perspective

## Story 6: 'Those pills are causing my rash!'

Beliefs are firmly held opinions, built upon individual experiences throughout our lives. They are usually bound by strong emotional responses, which is why most of us hold on to them even at times when logic says otherwise. So how do you manage your patients whose health beliefs contradict your own? Elsie reflects on a recent encounter with her GP.

> I was convinced my rash was caused by one of my pills. I'm not sure why I felt so strongly about this at the time, but I did. Perhaps I was influenced by what happened to one of my friends who come out in a nasty rash soon after starting a new tablet from her GP. Anyway, despite having been on my medications for years without any problems, and my doctor's alternative suggestion as to the cause, I was determined to stop it. Even though my GP didn't think it was going to make any difference, we agreed to give it a trial off this particular medication.
>
> My rash didn't get any better. In fact, it probably got a little worse. My doctor was lovely about it, though. Never once did she make me feel uncomfortable to share my views. I was certainly more open and willing to take her advice this time.
>
> Elsie, 81-year-old retired cleaner

We all have our own individual health beliefs. Doctors are no different. As patients, we do not always practise what we preach. Elsie firmly believed that she needed to stop one of her pills. Her GP disagreed but was able to manage their difference of opinion successfully. So much so, that Elsie now likes and trusts her GP more than ever before.

Showing respect for others' beliefs is crucial in the sharing process. This is rarely achieved by telling someone 'You are wrong!' We must be careful in our use of language when expressing an opinion. It will determine how we are perceived, and affect our chances of persuading others to come round to our way of thinking.

Be careful when using definitive statements to express your views. This can make your opinion sound like fact and risks closing off any further discussion (e.g. *'This pill is not causing your rash'*). Instead, consider a more open and diplomatic style. The use of 'I' statements can be effective here (e.g. *'I understand why you may believe that, but in my opinion I do not think the pills are the cause'*).

As with many things in life, dealing with people is less concerned with whether someone is right or wrong, and more about feelings and a shared desire to understand each other. Our patients will come with their preconceived ideas and expectations. Embrace them. Remain open and share yours.

# Key points

Sharing is the fourth 'S' in our model. It utilises all the relevant information gathered from earlier in the consultation and enables both the patient and doctor to have an open exchange of opinions as to what should happen next. It is an active decision-making process that allows the patient to shoulder some of the responsibility for any action plans. It involves sharing in the risk of any action or inaction and recognises any uncertainty that comes with that.

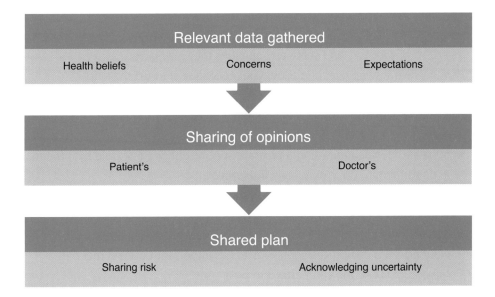

Once a shared plan has been agreed, then we can move into the final phase of the doctor–patient encounter – that of 'Securing' – ensuring that the consultation concludes safely.

## COMMUNICATION EXERCISE: practising Sharing

Choose a clinical encounter with a patient where there was a difference of opinion.

*Part 1*:    Pair up and tell your story to a colleague (or a bigger group, if you prefer). Include why you believe this difference of opinion occurred. Was there resolution? If so, what do you think helped? Is there anything you would do differently in similar circumstances?

*Part 2*:    Your colleague(s) should now ask you questions to clarify any aspects of the story and share any opinions they may have.

*Part 3*:    Now swap over and allow your colleague(s) to tell their story.

Alternative scenarios to consider rehearsing with another colleague could include:

- 50-year-old male requesting a prostate-specific antigen test; told by a friend a 'good thing to do'; completely fit and well
- 40-year-old female requesting the combined oral contraceptive; heavy smoker and refuses to give up
- 36-year-old male with a 1-day cough and runny nose; well otherwise; wanting antibiotics in case gets worse; has important business meeting at the end of week and can't afford to be ill
- 67-year-old female requesting oral hormone replacement therapy for first time.

Take turns being the doctor and the patient. Focus on sharing each other's knowledge, beliefs, concerns, expectations and, ultimately, risk.

# 5

# Securing

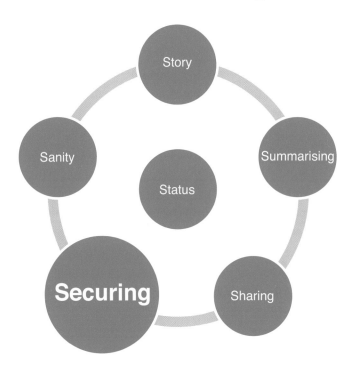

*There is no question that we must do more to secure our borders
– but how we go about securing them is also important.*

Mark Udall

*Security is, I would say, our top priority because for all the exciting
things you will be able to do with computers – organizing your
lives, staying in touch with people, being creative – if we don't
solve these security problems, then people will hold back.*

Bill Gates

# What is Securing?

Securing is defined as 'making secure' or safe and, in the context of a consultation, this relates to all the processes that help ensure any risks of harm are minimised as much as possible.

'Securing' the consultation is essential for safe medical practice. Risk will always exist in the medical profession, be it due to action or inaction. The aim of any advice, investigation or treatment is to help our patients, but, despite our best efforts, outcomes can be unpredictable and unfavourable. As mentioned in the previous chapter, GPs need to become adept at dealing with uncertainty. Uncertainty carries risk – should we act or watch and wait? If we act, can we do any harm? What are the potential consequences of inaction? Doctors make these decisions with almost every patient they see. Involving the patient and sharing this burden can help.

Each patient encounter will have its own unique set of factors that will influence the level of risk. For example, giving advice and managing a young child with a fever may differ slightly if this is mum's first child, compared with another mum who has two older children at home and has previous experience. Or consider advice given to a patient following a suspected minor head injury – your advice may depend on whether this person lives alone or whether there are other family cohabiting who can keep an eye open for any complications.

There are three stages to consider when assessing and managing risk.
1. **Identify** – what are the possible risks?
2. **Analyse** – how likely are they to be realised?
3. **Manage** – what strategies can be put in place to minimise these risks?

In this chapter, we will **explore various strategies for managing these risks and securing our consultations**.

# Story 1: Telephone consulting

How comfortable are you in managing concerns and queries from patients over the phone? How much of a difference does it make if you know the patient well? Rachel has recently registered at a new GP practice and recalls one of her first encounters there.

> I was really impressed with our new doctor. Although I've yet to meet him, he phoned me back after I rang for advice about my ongoing cough. I have had asthma for many years and it's not unusual in the winter months for it to play up. I was worried I needed something more than just my usual inhalers. I appreciate that there's only so much they can do over the phone. Anyway, he listened to what I had to say, asked a few more questions about how I was feeling and what I was currently using and arranged for a review with himself later in the week. I was very clear what the plan was and knew that someone would see me urgently before then if I got worse. I didn't think I would come off the phone feeling so reassured, but I did.
>
> Rachel, 37-year-old accountant

Managing risk steps up to a whole new level when consulting on the telephone. The absence of visual signs and cues increases the chances of misunderstanding between doctor and patient. Important diagnoses are more likely to be missed unless we 'secure' these encounters effectively. Rachel has had a positive experience with her GP over the phone. But what exactly has her doctor done to make her feel so reassured? It would appear from her story that listening, asking pertinent questions and setting up a clear plan that was acceptable to both parties were key. This involves setting out very clearly what to do if things get worse or do not go as expected.

Safety-netting is well recognised in many industries and professions, especially where risk exists. It was Roger Neighbour (*The Inner Consultation*) who brought a wider recognition of this concept to the medical consultation.[3] He suggests that we ask ourselves these three questions:

1. If I'm right, what do I expect to happen?
2. How will I know if I'm wrong?
3. What would I do then?

These are useful points to consider with all clinical encounters, as safety-netting is an essential component of Securing.

Another factor not to underestimate, especially on the phone, is that of empathy. Our empathy helps our patients feel understood and listened to, which in turn leads to greater trust and subsequent compliance with any management plan. Choose your words carefully and recognise that the tone of your voice and the rate and volume of your speech will all have an impact in achieving this (as discussed in Chapter 1: Status). Whatever is decided, it is important that both patient and doctor feel comfortable with the outcome. If you can't resolve an issue over the phone, is a face-to-face encounter required?

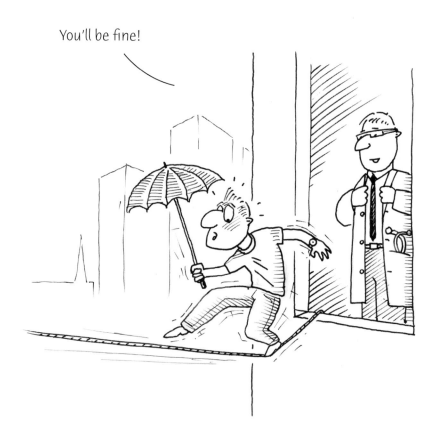

# Story 2: Home visits

For many doctors, home visits are a mixed bag. They can be challenging both clinically and socially but they can also be time-consuming. However, there is often rich information and insights that can be gained from assessing someone in his or her own home or natural environment that is not so readily available within a practice or clinic. Andrew reflects on a recent case involving a locum GP and an elderly patient, highlighting some of the additional challenges that home visits confer.

It was an unfortunate sequence of events, which has led to a significant change in our practice. A locum GP was helping us out for the day, whilst a couple of other doctors were on an update course. There were quite a few visits that morning and we asked our locum to see what appeared to be a relatively straightforward case – an elderly 87-year-old man with a chesty cough. He lived alone and rarely attended the surgery. His daughter, who lived about 30 miles away, had rung that morning to request the visit.

It was about 6 weeks later that the surgery was contacted again by the daughter. She was really angry and upset. Her father had collapsed the previous day and been admitted to hospital. He had a severe anaemia and a suspicious 'shadow' on his chest X-ray. She wanted to know why the GP practice had not picked up on this before.

What we discovered, was that the locum GP had prescribed antibiotics for a suspected chest infection, but had also noted how pale and cachectic he looked and had arranged for a district nurse to do some blood tests. The results had been seen by the registered GP, who picked up on a low haemoglobin, and asked our admin team to contact the patient to discuss further. After several attempts to contact the patient by phone, a message was left on his answering machine to call the surgery back. But he never did.

Since then, we have examined how we allocate, manage and feed back about our home visits. We hope now that there are better and safer systems in place to ensure any relevant follow-up occurs and what we will do if patients are not contactable.

Andrew, GP

Home visits are generally reserved for the most frail and vulnerable adults in our society. Physical or mental impairments may make them more reliant on others to help and represent them. 'Securing' these encounters can provide the doctor with additional challenges compared with the ones in a booked consultation within the practice.

Normally our patients take the initiative to report when they are not well and to chase results. It is not clear from Andrew's story who was left responsible for the ongoing follow-up of this elderly man and it raises many questions about all those involved.

- *The patient*. Did he understand why blood was being taken? Was he in a fit state to comprehend what the locum doctor advised? Did he have the practice's phone number to call back? Does he know how to use an answering machine? Can he hear properly?
- *The daughter*. What is her role in all this? She made the initial call. How much was she involved during the home visit and after? Did she know about the doctor's concerns?
- *The locum GP*. How clear was he with the patient about any follow-up? Did he check the patient's understanding? Had he left any written instructions for the patient or daughter? What safety netting did he have in place, considering that the patient lived alone? Did he hand over to any of the other GPs in the practice?
- *The practice*. What systems are in place to manage abnormal results? What happens when patients are not directly contactable? Should someone have called the daughter when the patient did not answer his phone?

We would need to speak to the locum doctor to discover what actually happened during the home visit, but what is clear is that responsibility needs to be shared. How we communicate and share the risks of any treatment or action plan will influence how outcomes are perceived by all involved. The medical profession has moved away from a paternalistic approach to healthcare, to one where patients are encouraged and empowered to make more of the decisions relating to themselves. Doctors continue to give their expert advice and opinion but, ultimately, it is our patients who decide whether they will be compliant or not. For those who, through illness or impairment, are unable to make such high-level decisions, then it becomes even more important that others involved in their care (e.g. family, carers, district nurses, community matron) are clear as to what is expected and what to do if things don't go according to plan.

# Story 3: The use of 'time'

It was Hippocrates who once said 'Healing is a matter of time but it is sometimes also a matter of opportunity'. How often are you aware of using time with your patients? What opportunities can this bring to your consultations and subsequently? Ivan, a GP trainer, shares with us why he believes that 'the use of time' is an essential part of a doctor's toolkit.

> It was just after I had decided to enter general practice, when a friend joked that I needed to get used to saying 'take two paracetamol, and come back in 2 weeks if you're not better!' If only that were more true. Whilst I still see the occasional 'cold' and sprain, most of my surgeries are full of chronic disease, mental health issues or complex elderly patients with multiple problems. And most of them do reliably return, and two paracetamol rarely satisfies!
>
> However, the use of time is a skill that I have come to appreciate more and more. It's one of my biggest assets as a GP. I use it for both diagnostic and therapeutic purposes and when I safety-net towards the end of my consultations. It is a skill that I try to encourage early on with my GP trainees, where feeling one has managed a case 'safely' remains a major concern.
>
> Ivan, GP trainer

Ivan's friend makes a joke that many of us have heard before in some shape or form. Within it, though, lies a large grain of truth: many people who visit their GP have a self-limiting illness that will resolve without the need for any medical intervention. Time and reassurance are what they need. Giving a time frame for patients to use as a rough guide to improvement can be very empowering for them in managing their symptoms, as well as allowing them 'permission' to return if they don't get better.

The actual face-to-face time doctors have with their patients is very short. A single consultation provides a brief view of an individual at a single point in their lives. Monitoring how symptoms and signs change (or not) over time can be extremely helpful in deciding what can be done next. Are they getting better? Or worse? Or much the same? Many doctors advocate the use of diaries to help patients monitor their symptoms – for example, with intermittent headaches or cyclical abdominal pains. Engaging our patients more in the diagnostic process may in turn lead to greater understanding and compliance with any subsequent treatment or management.

None of this is rocket science, but there is an art in knowing how to use time skilfully. If patients are going to place their trust in the use of time, then they need to understand your reasoning. How much time do you allow before deciding on any follow-up? What do you expect the patient to do during a period of observation? Are further tests (e.g. bloods) really necessary? The answers to these questions will vary depending on the problem you are trying to manage, but unless you actively think about them, and are clear with yourself and your patient, then you risk increasing the levels of uncertainty and worry rather than reducing them.

# Story 4: 'I can't get through to my GP!'

How easy do you find it to contact your GP? How quickly can you get hold of another colleague working in a different practice or hospital to discuss a particular case? How long would you be willing to wait to get through? Two minutes? Five? Ten? Most of us have waited at least that long trying to speak to someone at our bank or insurance company. It is hard to forget that feeling of frustration when you have been holding on, not knowing how much longer it will be before your call is answered. Mark describes the impact that his GP surgery's phone system has had on him.

> I have only one criticism about my GP practice, and that is the phones! I don't understand why it takes so long to get through to speak to someone. And I'm not just referring to the early morning rush when the phone lines first open. No matter what time of the day you call, it's a 10-minute wait, minimum! It must put a lot of people off.
>
> A couple of months ago, my GP arranged some blood tests and advised that I call back for the results. I still don't know what they are, as I've given up trying to get through. It's a real shame, as all the doctors, nurses and other staff who work there are really lovely. The building is relatively new and modern, and they run all sorts of extra clinics and services. You can even book appointments online. But their phone system is a nightmare.
>
> Mark, 40-year-old lawyer

Mark's practice may have high-calibre clinicians and a lovely working environment, but it is let down significantly by its poor accessibility to patients via the phone. A surgery's phone system is the main source of contact for our patients. Yet in Mark's case, the phone system has become a barrier to his ongoing healthcare. This becomes an even greater issue for those more acutely unwell and requiring more urgent advice.

It is common practice for GPs to advise their patients to call up for results of investigations, and in certain cases to inform their GP of current progress, especially if their symptoms worsen. The use of the phone can be a very useful tool in the 'safety-netting' process following a consultation. If it isn't, then ask yourselves why. This is where patient feedback questionnaires can prove instrumental in improving systems that are inadequate. Are there too few telephonists working at

Mark's practice for the demands of its population? Or is the phone system archaic and in desperate need of updating? Whatever the reason, it needs to be addressed to facilitate healthcare rather than hindering it.

# Story 5: 'How much do I need to record?'

Deciding how much to document following a consultation is very much down to individual professional judgement. Ideally, medical records will contain all the relevant information to allow doctors and healthcare professionals to facilitate ongoing advice and care, where they or others may or may not have been involved previously. There are also important medico-legal reasons why good documentation is essential. Ben works in several different practices and shares his views on this topic.

> One of the biggest challenges for me when I started my GP training was getting to grips with the computer system. It's quite a leap from the paper-based records used in most hospitals. It took me several weeks to feel comfortable using it and even now when I work in a practice which uses a different system to the one I trained with, it makes for a more demanding day. I'm not the quickest at typing, although I am gradually speeding up. I still need to give myself a minute or two at the end of each consultation to write up what happened. Not always easy when you are running late.
>
> There's a real variety between doctors as to how much they write. As a locum, most of the patients I see are a one-off. I'm aware that other doctors who see them later are relying on what I document to help with any further follow-up. For me, it's actually more about peace of mind. I know that any child who presents with a simple 'cold' could go on to develop meningitis and meningococcal septicaemia later that day. I write more for these cases than probably anything else. What I document is ultimately my biggest defence should any criticism about my clinical practice come my way.
>
> Ben, GP locum

We live in a litigious world and the stakes are rarely higher than when dealing with people's health and lives. This fact alone will motivate many doctors to keep good records. However, we would like to believe that all medical professionals see keeping good records as part of good medical practice, aiding communication between colleagues and ultimately facilitating our patients' ongoing care.

To save time, it can be very tempting to write very little and move onto your next patient. In the longer term, should there be any queries about what happened, or complaints, good documentation is likely to save you more than just time. Doctors see many patients in a single day, and it can be very difficult to recall, and prove, exactly what occurred with one particular patient, unless there is evidence to back this up. It is worth checking with your medical defence organisation what advice and guidance they offer. If you have ever had need to use them about a specific clinical case, then you will know that one of the first things they will ask for is what has been recorded. Note-keeping is our biggest asset here.

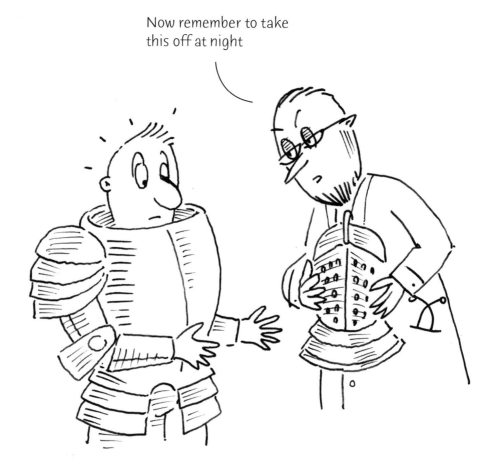

# Story 6: The challenges of working part-time

How many sessions a week do you work? What would you describe as full-time now? What systems are in place to look after your patients when you are not available? Annie, a part-time GP, describes how she has managed to make a more flexible working pattern work for herself and her practice.

> I have worked as a part-time GP for the last 10 years. I have four children, my youngest is still at nursery, and my oldest has just started secondary school. I don't know how I squeeze everything in, but I do, and I'm lucky my practice supports me in working 3 days each week. For most of my patients, this works fine, but there are a few who need advice and help on the days I'm not in. I've learnt not to feel guilty about this, as I do the best I can. I suppose it's no different at weekends or when doctors go on holiday. Most of our patients have come to accept that sometimes they will need to see another doctor, who may not be their preferred choice. As I don't work on Thursdays and Fridays, I try to hand over to my colleagues any relevant cases each Wednesday. As a general rule, we try to meet for a few minutes at midday, each day, to discuss and share any issues or concerns. This works really well and allows me to switch off from work when I'm not there.
>
> Annie, part-time GP

Part-time working patterns are commonplace now, especially in medicine. The sessional basis of general practice, in particular, allows doctors to have more flexibility in juggling work, family and other interests. As a natural consequence though, continuity of care for our patients may be threatened. So how can we minimise this risk?

For Annie, it is the process of regular 'handover'. She wants to know that her more vulnerable patients will be cared for when she is not there. Obviously, GPs cannot hand over every patient they see, but for those carefully selected cases that may require the assistance of other colleagues, such as those receiving 'end-of-life' care, it can have a significant impact on the quality of care that is given and perceived by all those involved. For the doctors, it is also likely to minimise any additional anxiety that may be caused by dealing with an unfamiliar case. After all, handover involves the sharing of responsibility for the care of our patients, which has obvious implications for patient safety, as well as professional protection for the clinician. If this is done badly, or not done at all, it risks misunderstanding and potential harm. This is particularly pertinent to colleagues who work shifts within hospital settings, although the principles of managing transitions of care apply to all medical specialties. The General Medical Council and medical defence organisations have clear guidance on this.

Clear and detailed documentation of clinical encounters, as illustrated in our previous story, is essential. As patient access has become more immediate, the choice of doctor has been restricted. Part-time working patterns for doctors emphasise this issue. Many patients now expect follow-up to be with another clinician and what we record may be the only formal handover we give to our next colleague who sees the same patient.

# Key points

Securing is the fifth 'S' in our model. It focuses on ensuring a safe conclusion to our patient encounters. How we manage risk will be influenced by individual patient and doctor factors, as well as the practice systems in place. A shared plan that includes clear safety-netting advice will help to empower our patients (and carers or families) to manage their health more effectively in the future. Sharing responsibility also provides more peace of mind for the doctor. Contemporaneous records and appropriate handover to colleagues secures the evidence after our consultations and provides a valuable resource for future care.

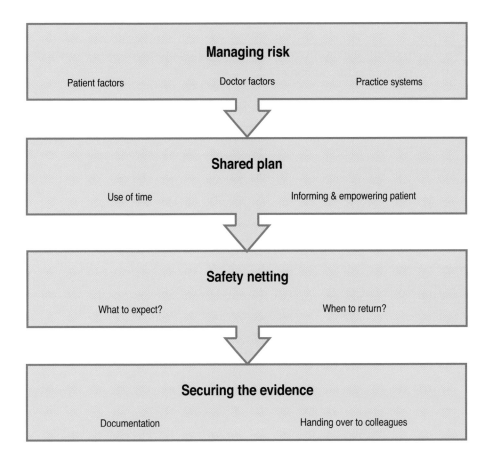

## COMMUNICATION EXERCISE: practising Securing

Choose a clinical encounter with a patient where a high level of uncertainty was involved. This uncertainty may have been because of diagnostic or therapeutic reasons, or both. Explore with a colleague (or group, if you prefer) what the risks were, and how you managed them.

Alternative scenarios to consider, rehearse and discuss could include:

- a young child with high fever
- a 50-year-old man with rectal bleeding
- a 2-hour history of right lower abdominal pain and loss of appetite
- end-of-life care.

Review any recent significant events. What Securing processes were in place (or not) that resulted in the outcomes?

# 6
# Sanity

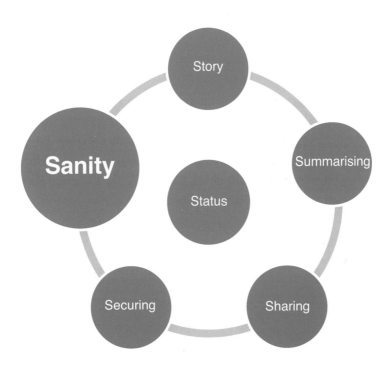

*When you get to the end of your rope, tie a knot and hang on.*

Franklin D Roosevelt

*'Inside every sane person there's a madman struggling to get out,' said the shopkeeper. 'That's what I've always thought. No one goes mad quicker than a totally sane person.'*

Terry Pratchett, *The Light Fantastic*

## What is Sanity?

According to the *Oxford Dictionary, Thesaurus and Wordpower Guide*,[4] when we are not maintaining our sanity, the faculties of reason, rationality, stability, lucidity and wits are in danger of disappearing. The same publication also tells us that when sanity prevails, wisdom, prudence, judiciousness, soundness and sensibleness abound.

> *Insanity: doing the same thing over and over again and expecting different results.*
>
> Albert Einstein

This quote is most apt in the world of medicine. Much of a doctor's workload is repetitive, yet each case requires meticulous and careful consideration, often under intense time pressures. If we are concerned about preserving our sanity but carry on regardless and change nothing in our routines, then the insanity Einstein talked about may arise. How we interact with our patients and colleagues will have a significant bearing on our sense of well-being. Embracing the five other Ss is therefore a crucial component of Sanity. If we consult well, we feel better ourselves.

In this chapter **we will identify the dangers and pitfalls, both mental and emotional, of working with a heavy caseload, and we will suggest a number of strategies and techniques to cope, and remain healthy in mind and body**.

# Dialogue 1: What puts you under pressure?
# (Dr Alex Watson interviewed by David Gillespie)

Dave   *Alex, I'm interested to know what threatens your sanity at work. As a doctor, what puts you under pressure?*

Alex   *I think it's the enormous amount of work we have and the relatively short amount of time we have to do it in. The day job has really intensified over the last few years and is not showing any signs of letting up. Our workload has been compressed. We constantly find ourselves running late ... running behind and that takes its toll. It's a much more intense day than it used to be. We're all feeling that burnout might be around the corner.*

Dave   *What are the factors that make you run late? What takes up the time and adds to the pressure?*

Alex   *So many things. Patient demand ... patient expectation ... A patient can have a shopping list with multiple agendas all raised in a single appointment. Then there can be complex cases, sometimes elderly patients with difficult pathology and chronic disease ... heavy emotional cases with mental illness ...*

Dave   *What about interruptions? Are you constantly being interrupted?*

Alex   *No ... not constantly, but it happens. People need to know things ... receptionists, colleagues ... and it all takes time.*

Dave   *So, do you get a bit of time to catch your breath in between patients?*

Alex   *Hardly. The in-between patient time is usually taken up with the interruptions or reading the next patient's notes.*

Dave   *So there's no switch off time?*

Alex   *Not as such ... no. But if there is an opportunity to regroup, switch off ... whatever you want to call it, we really should be grabbing it. It's crazy when you think about it ... most other jobs wouldn't have that kind of pressure. This is a job where we really have to concentrate, and if concentration is broken it can be hard to get it back.*

Dave   *What about the emotional impact? I mean ... people must be bringing in all sorts of emotions attached to their problems or their concerns and worries. How do you deal with that?*

| Alex | *You're right, they do and it can be very difficult. They might be scared, they might be tearful or even aggressive and angry . . . it's not easy.* |
|------|---|
| Dave | *No . . . as long as it doesn't turn you to the bottle, Alex. Mind you, they say that if you drink less than your doctor you're probably okay. Is that right?* |
| Alex | *No comment!* |
| Dave | *Sorry, that was a bit cheeky! But seriously, it's not just you is it? Your colleagues are dealing with all that emotion as well. Do you have some sort of support network for each other or does everyone just get on with it by themselves?* |
| Alex | *Well, yes and no. Of course that's what should happen but it's not always the case. And then you can have difficult colleagues and staff to deal with . . . it's just like any other business in that respect. Believe me, there are some days when you just can't wait to get home!* |
| Dave | *When you get home can you switch off? How good are you at leaving it in the locker . . . do you chill well or do you take it home?* |
| Alex | *I'm not bad. My wife is a GP so she understands. We try hard to park our work and concentrate on the family as much as we can. In fact, listening to what sort of day our children have had can be really calming and distracting from any stressful situations we've been dealing with.* |
| Dave | *Okay, Alex, business aside . . . I've often wondered how you relax out of surgery hours. What happens in the private life of Dr Watson?* |
| Alex | *Mind your own business.* |

# Dialogue 2: Perspective and confidence (interview with Dr Chris Shambrook)

To help us with this chapter on sanity, we decided to talk to two experts in the fields of well-being and self-preservation while working in a high-pressure environment on a daily basis. Our first conversation was with Dr Chris Shambrook, psychologist to the Great Britain Rowing Team since 1997 and Performance Director at K2, a high-performance consultancy firm. We asked Chris what he thought are the principal components of maintaining our sanity. He said quite simply that they are **perspective** and **confidence**. Here is what he had to say on these subjects.

## Perspective

Maintaining a healthy perspective on everything we do is vitally important for success and I think what you guys say about 'Sharing' is spot on. Sharing can really help. We need to be checking in with ourselves on a regular basis. Making sure we have a balanced view of the world. Making sure we're not losing perspective.

It's important to have a baseline and that we don't go too far from it. If we wander off we begin to focus on the demand we have and how large it is, rather than the quality of the tools we have and the superb talent and support we have from others to meet the demand . . . this only results in a loss of energy.

No one should try to be an island. In fact I think supervision ought to be part of a doctor's performance . . . sharing caseloads . . . comparisons . . . talking things through . . . letting off stress and pressure for survival and sanity. I really do believe that creating a non-hierarchical network of clinical supervision is the way forward . . . mutual support in a proactive way can be a tremendous help for everyone.

Another important aspect of a healthy perspective is being able to park stuff and move on. By that I mean refocus and not carry baggage from one consultation to the next. Hard to do sometimes, but so important. It's what really great golfers do so well. If they have a bad hole, they don't allow themselves to carry that emotion it gave them or any negativity to the next one. We are all capable of finding personal routines that allow us to remain focused on the moment. It's about having a controlled engagement with the environment, rather than a roller-coaster ride of 'how do I get through it?' ... and asking ourselves questions like '... am I making a proper transition from work to home? Do I have a clear plan for the next morning?'

I also think it's important to rest, recover and refuel properly. It's vital that we eat well and that the body enjoys the downtime we give it, so it is acting in a restorative way rather than a coping way. There's a big difference.

## Confidence

You need to have a solid, contemporary picture of yourself ... be aware and value all the strengths you have and never take them for granted, because they are the cornerstone of your ability to deal with your caseload. You must look at your whole profile as a performer and ask questions like 'how successful has today been?' ... rather than 'did I just get through it?' ... and share those successes. Relate them back to supervision.

You have to ask yourself 'what are the inevitable scenarios I am going to face given that I have chosen to venture into this field of work?' ... and 'what are the abilities and talents I have to deal with them?' Thinking like this will help you make your implicit knowledge explicit.

The things you say in your first chapter about getting the right level of status are key to being confident. If the practice or organisation you work in encourages mutual support, then it is more likely that the individuals within it will flourish. Being able to connect well and be trusted and liked is a real confidence giver.

So, in summary, **perspective** relates to worrying about the right stuff at the right time, rather than globally worrying about everything. **Confidence** is part of our toolbox, which enhances our perceived ability to cope and manage our workload effectively.

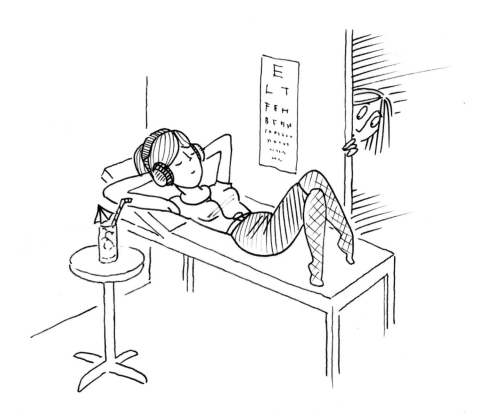

## Dialogue 3: Looking after ourselves and preventing 'burnout' (interview with Dr Tim Anstiss)

Our second interview was with Dr Tim Anstiss – a doctor, lecturer and coach with an interest in health and well-being. Our main focus was on preventing 'burnout'. Tim highlighted five key areas to consider:

1. clarifying values and strengths
2. problem-solving and being assertive
3. learning to relax and cultivating mindfulness
4. developing and maintaining balance
5. knowing when to seek help.

Here is what Tim had to say on these issues.

> There are a number of strategies we can develop to take better care of ourselves, especially when we are working hard in often stressful circumstances. Being **clear about our values** is a big part of maintaining sanity and can help us keep things in perspective. What do we feel strongly about? What is our idea of happy living? How far might we have strayed from that? Exploring and finding ways to **use our strengths** in our work and wider lives can also aid resilience and well-being. But first you might need to get a better understanding of what your strengths are, and there are various online tools and surveys that can help you identify these. If we lose our sense of what is important to us and who we are, then loss of meaning and purpose may follow.
>
> I think **problem solving** is another skill to get better at. Making a list of problems and issues to be addressed – and important things to get done – is something we should do regularly. Then, of course, we need to prioritise and take action. **Being assertive** and able to communicate openly will also make you more effective and may improve your well-being, even if you don't get the result you want. Of course, there will be things you cannot change. It was the American theologian Reinhold Niebuhr who originally said:
>
>> . . . grant me the serenity to accept the things I cannot change, the courage to change the things I can, and wisdom to know the difference.

Another important ability to develop is **how to bring on the relaxation response**. When the body is relaxed it is harder for the mind to be stressed. There are body to mind techniques that bring about a state of relaxation, such as exercise, progressive muscular relaxation, taking a bath, having sex … though probably not all at the same time! Then there are the mind to body techniques such as meditation and **mindfulness**. My favourite book on this subject is *Mindfulness* by Professor Mark Williams and Dr Danny Penman,[5] with a CD-ROM and a series of 10-minute exercises to practise.

Mindfulness and relaxation can help you stay calm and centred, in touch with the present moment and may also help to improve the conversations you have with patients, colleagues and family members. Then there's motivational interviewing, which encourages a more gentle and guiding style of consulting, rather than a telling and instructing style, which risks triggering resistance and defensiveness. This can help you avoid conflict and reduce your experience of negative emotions.

Developing and maintaining interests and hobbies outside of your working life, or even acquiring a specialism within your work, may help prevent burnout. Play a sport, do some exercise, spend more time in contact with nature, go to the movies or the theatre, learn to cook better – all these things help us to stay human and **balanced**.

And if we are really troubled or struggling, it may be appropriate **to seek help** and talk to someone – perhaps a trained professional – to help us get back on track and recover lost well-being.

All these strategies and skills can help us develop resilience, to recover, protect and improve our well-being. We owe it to ourselves to be rounded human beings, connected and engaged in a life of meaning and purpose … flourishing and thriving whilst doing our best for others.

# Dialogue 4: Maintaining focus (David Gillespie interviewed by Dr Alex Watson)

Alex  *Okay, Dave, here's a question for you. How can your world . . . the world of theatre, advise my world of medical consultation on keeping sane and remaining focused?*

Dave  *That's a good question. I think that our worlds are similar in some ways.*

Alex  *Really? You sure?*

Dave  *Yes. We both have to give a fresh and spontaneous performance for everyone that comes to see us . . . and I suppose that means being able to refocus time after time to do it. Each new consultation for you is a new performance for me. Maybe the closest comparison could be the two shows in 1 day situation or even three if it's pantomime season . . . each audience has to be given the same degree of enthusiasm and energy that the last audience received.*

Alex  *I think I'm with you. Go on.*

Dave  *Well . . . in a broad sense a new audience each night in the theatre deserves my full focus and concentration, in the same way each patient deserves yours. In a more detailed sense, each scene an actor plays has to have the same degree of concentration as the next, which is probably getting closer to the kind of intensity that you guys have to work with.*

Alex  *Are you saying that we should look at each consultation as a scene in a play?*

Dave  *I don't know . . . maybe. Maybe it is a new scene, only you have a change of cast with every scene . . . apart from you being the central character, of course.*

Alex  *Ah . . . but there's a big difference, Dave: you get to rehearse your scenes . . . we don't have that luxury.*

Dave  *Yeah, okay . . . fair point. Or maybe you do to an extent.*

Alex  *This better be good.*

Dave  *I hope so. Rehearsed spontaneity is what we're talking about. It's a bit like what Chris Shambrook was saying. What are the pos-*

*sible scenarios I might encounter . . . and how would I respond to them? Whose Line Is It Anyway?*

Alex     *What?*

Dave     *The TV programme . . . Whose Line Is It Anyway?*

Alex     *Er . . . yes?*

Dave     *Well . . . those actors and comedians can't go on that programme unprepared. That kind of spontaneity has to have been considered in some way. What can possibly be thrown at me? What will be my response? It's the apparent freshness, focus and concentration they bring to it that lets them connect with their audience.*

Alex     *Okay. I see where you're coming from . . . but here's one for you. How do actors refocus between scenes and is there something doctors can get from that?*

Dave     *Ah . . . now this is where you guys draw the short straw. All sorts of thoughts and behaviours can be rehearsed. Actors still have to perform in the now and be totally focused on that moment in the same way that a doctor does in consultation, and be authentic. The difference is in the refocusing between the scenes. Actors get to rehearse the refocus because they know what scene is coming next . . . unless, of course, it's a completely improvised piece.*

Alex     *But a doctor's scenes are totally improvised. Yes, we may have been able to rehearse scenarios in our minds but how can we refocus for every consultation, day after day, week after week?*

Dave     *I think the fact that you have been able to prepare for most consultation scenarios must be a great help and has to be a support emotionally too. I guess the difficulty is not to carry any of those feelings to the next consultation and be able to approach it freshly. Perhaps this is what Tim Anstiss was saying about mindfulness and meditation. I know there isn't much time between appointments, but maybe there are some simple and quick things that can be done to help refocus the mind and keep the emotional status where it needs to be.*

Alex     *Like what?*

Dave     *Breathing exercises can be a great help to bring about calm, and might only take a minute . . . just focusing on the breathing mechanism and nothing else.*

| Alex | *Yes, I suppose that might be really helpful if the patient has been aggressive or confrontational. It would certainly help to bring the heart rate down.* |
| --- | --- |
| Dave | *Yeah . . . and clear the mind. Another technique would be to focus on something in the room . . . a picture . . . a photo . . . an object of some sort . . . then close your eyes and try to remember every colour, shape and detail . . . focusing on nothing else but that task. Again this could take no more than a minute or two.* |
| Alex | *Okay.* |
| Dave | *Or a similar technique could be to hold an object . . . close the eyes and focus on how that object feels and describe it aloud . . . but giving total focus to that.* |
| Alex | *Sounds simple.* |
| Dave | *Yes . . . it should be. Maybe another go at a clue in a crossword . . . a minute of sudoku . . . or a quick look at an article in a medical paper or journal.* |
| Alex | *And failing that?* |
| Dave | *Drugs.* |
| Alex | *Stop it!* |
| Dave | *Sex.* |
| Alex | *Now you've gone too far.* |
| Dave | *Rock and Roll?* |
| Alex | *Hmm . . . okay . . . but not in that order.* |

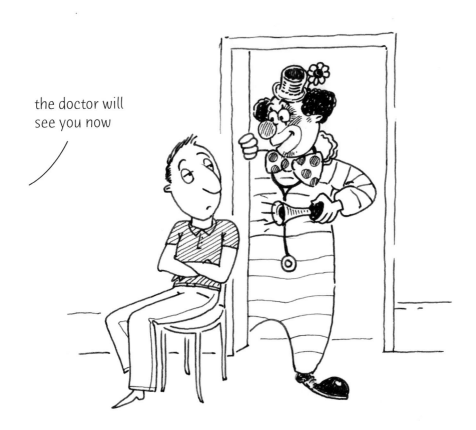

the doctor will
see you now

# Dialogue 5: Putting theory into practice (Alex and Dave)

Alex      *There's a lot of great advice, but knowing and doing are two different things!*

Dave      *That's very true. So why don't you start by making a list of the things that might help you throughout your working day? Start from the moment you wake up in the morning, to the moment you go to bed.*

Alex      *Okay, here it goes . . .*

*Before work – Have a proper unhurried breakfast.*

*Arrive at work early – If I get in early, then I can clear some of my paperwork whilst still with a fresh mind. I slow down later in the day, and these tasks take much longer.*

*Start morning surgery as early as possible – This takes the pressure off later in the morning, when home visits and other meetings are scheduled. It may also mean I get a few more minutes to eat lunch in peace.*

*Consider adequate 'catch-up' slots – I tend to overrun with certain patients (e.g. elderly, chronic disease, mental health), and I hate it when I'm running really late. It all adds up, every extra couple of minutes here and there. There's also this strange phenomenon that patients who are generally seen on time are more likely to respect the allocated time, whereas those whom have been kept waiting longer seem more reluctant to leave. Perhaps some feel that instead of coming back another time to discuss a separate issue, they will try their luck and raise it then, thereby avoiding the hassle of another long wait? I tend to finish my surgeries at a similar time each day, regardless of what time my last patient is booked in. So why not put in the relevant 'catch-up' slots needed?!*

*Temporary 'alerts' on the booking system for complex patients – If there are patients who are going to take twice as long as others, such as the very frail and elderly with poor mobility, and those with multiple problems, then a longer or double appointment may be more appropriate. An alert on the booking system is useful for our receptionists when making the appointment.*

***Reducing interruptions*** *– It's a big enough challenge to deal with all my patients booked in during surgery time, without interruptions from other colleagues, trainees and receptionists. There is only so much you can focus and concentrate on at the same time. I've heard that some practices have allocated times each day for their receptionists and administrative team to discuss any queries, rather than in between patient appointments. If additional clinical support is required on a regular basis by other colleagues, such as a new or struggling trainee doctor, then it is worth respecting the additional time needed to provide this, perhaps with additional 'catch-up/ training' slots.*

***Realistic patient expectations*** *– I wish some of my patients were more realistic about what is achievable within a single appointment. I appreciate it is not always convenient for them to take time off work or school to attend and so there is a temptation to save up all their concerns. Of course, some people may have more than one problem that is linked to the same cause, and we as doctors need to be able to discern what may be connected and what is not. However, the vast majority of people I see with 'lists' have very separate problems, and I want to deal with any concerns properly and safely. Generally one appointment allows me to deal with one main problem. We encourage our patients to book a longer/double appointment if they have more to discuss. We do try to highlight this in our waiting rooms, in an attempt to raise patient awareness.*

***Good team playing*** *– It makes such a big difference to my day when we are working well as a team. It's so easy to become isolated and overwhelmed with the volume of workload, especially during the busier winter months. I'm a great believer in regular contact and open communication to allow good practice to flourish and any frustrations or resentments to be aired and resolved. No one wants to work alongside a 'difficult' colleague. Most perceived problems are due to poor or inadequate communication. We need one another. We rely on one another.*

*Recognising and respecting that different colleagues have different ways of working* – *I am aware that my colleagues and I bring different skills and gifts to our practice. Appreciating these differences makes each individual feel valued. This is essential for ongoing team cohesion and job satisfaction.*

*Stop for lunch* – *It's tempting to press on through the day without stopping for lunch or hydrating. There's always something else that needs doing. My productivity improves significantly when I respect these basic needs, especially in the afternoon!*

*After work* – *It can be hard to switch off after the intensity that general practice demands. I try to do something physical, like running or swimming, at least twice a week. I enjoy music and support a choir. I need to relax and unwind before bedtime, otherwise I don't sleep well, and that's not a good start for the next working day!*

| | |
|---|---|
| Dave | *Well there you go, Alex. That's quite a list you've got there.* |
| Alex | *These are currently the main issues for me, which may change with time. I could have included a lot more. I didn't even mention spending time with my family and friends.* |
| Dave | *Yes, and we can often underestimate how important our nearest and dearest are to us, and us to them. Our sanity, or lack of, will impact on them too.* |
| Alex | *I do think doctors are becoming increasingly aware of maintaining a healthy work–life balance. I feel very fortunate still to be working as a doctor. It remains one of the most fulfilling careers out there.* |
| Dave | *In the words of Rudyard Kipling, so long as 'you can keep your head when all about you are losing theirs . . .!'* |

# Key points

Sanity is the sixth 'S' in our model. It is linked to our ability to embrace the first five Ss, because how we feel about our consultations with patients is likely to have a significant impact on our sense of well-being. Maintaining a healthy mind and body is essential in a profession where the stakes and pressures are consistently high and features of burnout are common. Addressing our basic physiological needs before, during and after work must not be underestimated, and these will affect our performance. We need to be aware of our own individual factors that put us under pressure and develop strategies to address these. If our perceived abilities to cope match or exceed the perceived demands, then we feel in a strong position. Effective teamwork, where important issues are regularly shared, will also support our confidence, as well as the organisation we work in.

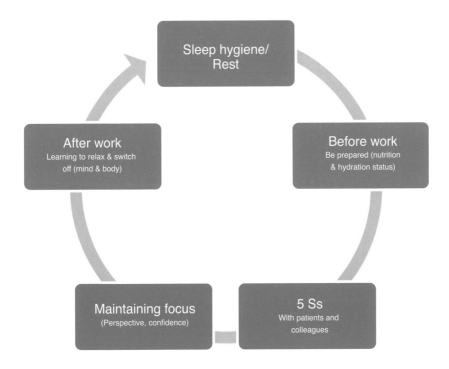

## COMMUNICATION EXERCISE: practising Sanity

### Breathing exercises

You can spend as little or as long as you like on these – before work, in between consultations, after work or just before going to bed. They are good for relaxation and will help to release tension.

- Breathe in for a count of seven and release on an 'sssss' for a count of 10.
- Repeat several times before increasing release counts in fives.
- We are looking for a fluid and constant release of air, which can be determined by the consistency of the 'S' sound.
- Repeat but releasing on a 'shhhh' sound – this is not as easy.
- These can be repeated as often as you like, with breaks in between each exercise so you do not hyperventilate.

### Group Sanity exercise

Snowball exercise – start on your own and make a list of what you do at work and outside to maintain your sanity. Then pair up and share with another colleague. Now get together with another pair (so a group of four now) and share again, and this time make a formal list that can then be shared with a larger group.

# Summary

We set out to write this book with the intention of creating a framework of communication that is immediately accessible and easy to apply. *Six S for Success* has been designed to do just that in the context of doctors' consultations with patients. We alluded briefly to a personal brand in our chapter on Story and we feel that it is appropriate to conclude this book with another look at the importance of our individual brand and the way it is perceived.

Visiting the doctor is an experience and if we can make that experience comfortable, bearable and even pleasant, our brand will be perceived in a favourable way. Experts will tell us that a brand is more than a logo or a motif, more than a design or a badge. They will tell us that it is the substance beneath that really matters. It is the experience we give to our clients or patients, the feeling they take away from that experience, and the story they tell about that experience. Naturally, we want that story to represent our service in a positive way.

The brand of our service must be lived by every part of our organisation, even by the tone and efficiency of our call-waiting facility, because that is where the experience begins and continues until we get to speak to a real person. It becomes an ensemble piece and it is important that the brand creators ensure that every team member, from front-of-house to GP to pharmacy, is striving for the same common goal.

Six S for Success is a template that is simple, easy to remember and built to last. It is there to support and underpin your confidence. If the Ss are strong, the brand is strong. Let it work for you.

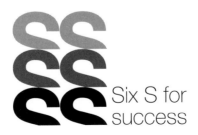

# References

1. Goleman D. *Emotional Intelligence: why it can matter more than IQ*. London: Bloomsbury Publishing; 1996.
2. Carnegie D. *How to Win Friends and Influence People*. New York, NY: Simon and Schuster; 1936.
3. Neighbour R. *The Inner Consultation: how to develop an effective and intuitive consulting style*. 2nd ed. Oxford: Radcliffe Publishing; 2005.
4. Soanes C, Hawker S, Waite M, editors. *Oxford Dictionary, Thesaurus and Wordpower Guide*. Oxford: Oxford University Press; 2001.
5. Williams M and Penman D. *Mindfulness*. London: Piatkus; 2011.

# Index

key points in 81
use of term 2, 68
self-preservation 87
sexuality 32, 47, 91, 94
Shambrook, Chris 87
sharing
    and agreement 56–7
    exercises in 66
    key points in 65
    and perspective 87
    of responsibility 61–2, 72, 79
    of successes 88
    of uncertainty 58
    use of term 2, 54
sick notes 61
six Ss 1–3
sleep hygiene 99
social abilities 17–18
spontaneity, rehearsed 92–3
status
    and confidence 88
    emotional 17–18, 93
    exercises on 20–1
    key points on 19
    physical 7–8, 12
    and story 35–6
    use of term 1–2, 6
    vocal 7, 14–16
story
    and cultural background 32–3
    disconnecting from 36
    eliciting full 30–1
    exercises for 38
    first minute of 26
    interrupting 29
    key points on 37
    listening to 28
    sharing 34–5, 66
    and summarising 51
    use of term 2, 24
stress 9, 41, 87

subtext 30–1, 37
summarising
    and complaints 43–4
    exercises in 51
    as interactive 47–8
    key points in 50
    and listening 41–2
    and multiple issues 46
    and third parties 45
    use of term 2, 40

teamwork 97–9
telephone
    giving advice over 25
    managing concerns over 69–70
    office systems of 75–6
    sending messages by 71
    summarising over 45
theatre 92–3
time, use of 73–4
tone, vocal 15–16

uncertainty
    managing 60
    and risk 68
    sharing 58
    and time 74

vocal exercises 21
voice
    appropriate 14–16
    muttering 7
    raising 9, 11
Voltaire 1
volume, vocal 16

work–life balance 98
worry
    and behaviour 12
    of patients 9, 47
    and time 74

## CPD with Radcliffe

You can now use a selection of our books to achieve CPD (Continuing Professional Development) points through directed reading.

We provide a free online form and downloadable certificate for your appraisal portfolio. Look for the CPD logo and register with us at: www.radcliffehealth.com/cpd

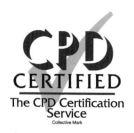